PENGUIN BOOKS

The Pioppi Diet

'This book is revolutionary. It should be read by everyone'
Sir Richard Thompson, Her Majesty
The Queen's personal physician 1984–2005 and
Past President of the Royal College Of Physicians

'A fearless and brilliant book that stands to dramatically
improve the nation's health'
Professor David Haslam, Chair, National Obesity Forum

'Changing lifestyles is essential to tackle the ailments of obesity
and this book is an articulate, common sense and practical way
of choosing wisely what you eat. It is a must have for every
household and a must read for every medical student and doctor'
Professor Dame Sue Bailey, Chair, Academy of Medical
Royal Colleges

'When delivering education for the prevention and management
of obesity and type-2 diabetes, I see immense benefits when
people adopt a real-food dietary approach eliminating refined
carbs and incorporating natural healthy fats. This book is a must
for anyone who wishes to improve their health'
Dr Trudi Deakin PhD, Chief Executive and Research
Dietician for X-Pert Health and founding member of the
Public Health Collaboration

'This brilliant book by Aseem Malhotra reinforces the
message that the obesity epidemic is eminently reversible and
provides clear, definitive, unambiguous information about
the key role of nutrition and lifestyle on the causation and
reversal of the chronic diseases plaguing the western world.
The pub

Pro

Essex County Council

3013021371926 2

'It is ridiculous that we treat diseases with a multitude of drugs that potentially can make patients even more ill without addressing the root cause. This superb ground-breaking book reveals that THE best MEDICINE is actually a HEALTHY LIFESTYLE AND HEALTHY NUTRITION'
Esther van Zuuren, MD, Methods Editor Cochrane Skin Group, Recommendations Editor Dynamed

'Cardiologist Dr Aseem Malhotra's lifestyle plan has the potential to reverse India's heart disease and type-2 diabetes epidemics. This book is a must read'
Kapil Dev, former Indian Cricket Captain

'I am more convinced every day that the nutrition principles contained in *The Pioppi Diet* are the key to improving our heath and reversing the devastating effects of chronic diseases such as type-2 diabetes and cardiovascular disease'
Professor Peter Brukner, Sports and Exercise Physician, Australian cricket team doctor

'Thankfully, over the last decade there has been an enormous backlash against the now defunct low-fat message. Dr Aseem Malhotra has been at the forefront of the push to move low-fat eating into the history book of medical mistakes. If society adopted the principles in Dr Malhotra's new book *The Pioppi Diet*, many cardiologists would be twiddling their thumbs due to lack of work'
Dr Ross Walker, Preventative Cardiologist, Sydney, Australia

'Aseem Malhotra's easily accessible book conveys a message which is of paramount importance for individual and public health: the way we live is a root cause of almost all non-communicable diseases we are faced with today. Using drugs as a primary means to restore the damage done is as ridiculous as trying to empty the ocean with a thimble'
Hanno Pijl, internist-endocrinologist, professor of Diabetology, Leiden University Medical Center, The Netherlands

'Modern society has lost its way in combining the best science and practice of nutrition and turning it into good health. At last here is your guide to getting back on track and helping us all live longer, better lives'
Grant Schofield PhD, Professor of Public Health Auckland University of Technology, Chief Advisor Health and Nutrition, New Zealand Ministry of Education

'An essential read that profiles the most powerful drug in the world: Lifestyle; spelled out in all its simplicities. Eat whole, unprocessed foods, increase movement, reduce stress and don't smoke to live a long, healthy life'
Caryn Zinn PhD, NZ Registered Dietitian and AUT Senior Lecturer

DR ASEEM MALHOTRA

Described as an 'inspiration' by Jamie Oliver, internationally renowned award-winning consultant cardiologist Dr Aseem Malhotra has become one of the most influential and well-known health campaigners in the UK. He writes regularly in academic medical journals and print newspapers such as the *Guardian*, the *Telegraph* and the *Daily Mail* and is regularly seen on broadcast media in his campaign against sugar and highlighting the harms of too much medicine.

Dr Malhotra has been named alongside anti-obesity activists such as Michael Bloomberg and Michelle Obama and was featured in the *New York Times* on his documentary film *The Big Fat Fix*, which in July 2016 premiered in British parliament and was also subsequently screened in the European Parliament. He is also the cardiologist advisor to the UK's National Obesity Forum. *The Pioppi Diet* is his first book.

DONAL O'NEILL

Donal O'Neill is an Irish born, independent documentary filmmaker. A former international track and field athlete, Donal's passion for health and human performance resonates throughout his films. In 2015 he joined forces with Dr Aseem Malhotra to make *The Big Fat Fix*. World renowned sports scientist Professor Tim Noakes has hailed it as 'the best health movie ever'.

The Pioppi Diet, co-written with Dr Malhotra, is Donal's first book.

@cerealkillers13
@facebook.com/cerealkillersmovie

The Pioppi Diet

DR ASEEM MALHOTRA
and
DONAL O'NEILL

PENGUIN BOOKS

PENGUIN BOOKS

UK | USA | Canada | Ireland | Australia
India | New Zealand | South Africa

Penguin Books is part of the Penguin Random House group of companies
whose addresses can be found at global.penguinrandomhouse.com.

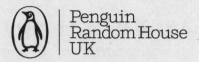

First published 2017
001

Copyright © Dr Aseem Malhotra and Donal O'Neill, 2017
Photography Copyright © Clare Winfield
Food Styling: Kat Mead
Prop Styling: Louie Waller

The moral right of the author has been asserted

Set in 12.5/14.75 pt Garamond MT Std
Typeset by Jouve (UK), Milton Keynes
Printed in Great Britain by Clays Ltd, St Ives plc

A CIP catalogue record for this book is available from the British Library

ISBN: 978–1–405–93263–9

www.greenpenguin.co.uk

MIX
Paper from
responsible sources
FSC® C018179

Penguin Random House is committed to a
sustainable future for our business, our readers
and our planet. This book is made from Forest
Stewardship Council® certified paper.

Aseem: *For my mother and father, Anisha and Kailash. Your abundance of love, kindness, honesty and integrity constantly inspires me to be a better person and a better doctor.*

Donal: *For my Godfather, Brian. It's not* Ulysses. *But you would have enjoyed the good news about red wine!*

Contents

Foreword by Professor David Haslam, Chair, National Obesity Forum

Being a renowned and popular interventional cardiologist is impressive, to be able to energetically communicate knowledge and skills over a wide range of written and broadcast media is even more notable, but to fearlessly broadcast controversial science which is not widely accepted by the public or the medical profession, despite being aware of the furore it will cause, is exemplary. This book is fearless, and takes religious dietetic dogma by the neck with both hands and gives it a severe shaking. It reveals why current backward thinking and dangerous teaching came about due to flawed research seventy years ago, and how the medical profession should hold up its hand, accept the blame for the current obesity epidemic, and make up for it by apologizing and shouting the correct message from the hilltops. There is nothing fanciful about the message or the science upon which this book is based. It relies on genuine and impeccable sources, and can be trusted implicitly.

There is increasing concern around the growing importance of not being overweight, obesity and type-2 diabetes globally. Einstein described the insanity of attempting the same failed solutions over and over again, hoping that they'll work next time; this encapsulates the direction in which academia and government are heading towards obesity management. Failed science needs to be questioned, not reinforced. The recent government Eatwell Guide is a case in point – a high-carbohydrate diet, which has played a major part in the obesity epidemic, has been reinforced by the amount of carbohydrate in a person's recommended daily consumption being increased. There comes a time when we need to scratch our collective heads and wonder what on earth is going on, and how we can change in order to reduce obesity levels and save countless lives. Studies dating back seventy years ostensibly shed doubt on ancient dietary guidelines. However, any scientific study needs to be questioned; this is the point of peer reviewing of academic papers. This book clearly states that, however ingrained nutritional concepts are, in the light of the continuing obesity epidemic we should be questioning and re-evaluating them. Famously, the first words a medical student hears at medical school are 'Half of what you learn here will be proved false in the future; the trouble is, we don't know which half.' Well, now we know a little bit about the false half: it is public health, government and dietetic dogma that is being proved to be erroneous, and it is up to fearless and skilled physicians like Aseem Malhotra to make some waves and overcome the views of dyed-in-the-wool traditionalists.

Hands up who knows what the Mediterranean Diet is? Well, think again. This brilliant book demonstrates the evolution of the concept 'diet', based on the ancient Greek meaning, referring to food, lifestyle and culture. Aseem Malhotra and Donal O'Neill trace the modern Mediterranean Diet back to its authors, Margaret and Ancel Keys, in a rather fond, nostalgic way, despite current scientific analysis demonstrating that much of Ancel's work was flawed. But the particularly enticing element is how southern Italian lifestyle and culture are woven into the plot, along with the romance of food and the relaxed frame of mind and body inherent to the people of this beautiful coastline. The Mediterranean Diet never looked so tempting, comprising locally, naturally sourced fish, meat, vegetables, olives and more. One used to have to move to the Med, but not anymore. Now, you can bring the Mediterranean Diet into your own kitchen and incorporate it into your lifestyle. There is so much that modern advice and guidelines could do to improve the nation's health, if it weren't for the paranoia of public health bosses and the intransigence of traditionalist physicians in failing to change their ways.

One of the last great and sensible medical textbooks was written in 1951 by Raymond Greene (the novelist Graham's brother). After this, falsehoods and misperceptions were peddled ubiquitously. Greene wrote, with regard to obesity:

Foods to be avoided:

1. Bread and everything else made with flour
2. Cereals, including breakfast cereal and milk puddings
3. Potatoes and all other white root vegetables

4. Foods containing much sugar
5. All sweets

You can eat as much as you like of the following foods:

1. Meat, fish, birds
2. All green vegetables
3. Eggs, dried or fresh
4. Cheese
5. Fruit, if unsweetened or sweetened with saccharin, except grapes and bananas.

This is the perfect advice for a healthy diet and to counteract obesity. The discarding of these excellent rules, and the total reversal by Public Health England, has underpinned the obesity epidemic over recent decades.

Science, and therefore clinical treatment, can advance only if clinicians such as Aseem Malhotra study the science behind current guidelines, question them, and change them as appropriate. This book is a fantastic example of a top clinician looking at himself in the mirror, realizing the faults of his profession and having the courage to blow the whistle, in the media, on what most doctors and nurses either misunderstand, or know to be true but feel unable to transmit to vulnerable patients.

Maybe the history of obesity will be defined by Hippocrates, Galen, Celsus, Sushruta, Maimonides, George Cheyne, Raymond Greene and Aseem Malhotra. If so, I will stand there beside him, supporting him in any way I can.

Aseem Malhotra is experienced enough to be able to

thoroughly assess the evidence surrounding diet and disease and thick-skinned enough to battle the slings and arrows that have inevitably followed him, but given his knowledge, his views, his research and his powers of communication, we may actually be able to look forward to a brighter future with regard to obesity and rates of preventable death. Congratulations, Aseem and Donal, on a fearless and brilliant book that stands to dramatically improve the nation's health.

Introduction

'It is health that is the real wealth, and not pieces
of gold and silver.'

– Mohandas K. Gandhi

As a qualified doctor for over fifteen years and a practising cardiologist who has treated thousands of patients in my career, including operating on hundreds with heart disease, I have come to realize that much of modern medical practice has become no better than putting a sticking plaster on a severed artery. For decades, our medical culture and resources have been misdirected towards treating the symptoms of disease and not directly tackling the root causes.

As a result of this failed model, healthcare is in crisis and we are all suffering. Over 60 per cent of the UK adult population are overweight or obese. More disturbingly, a third of children are in the same category by the time they leave primary school. And the trends are getting worse. The situation has become so grave that the UK's chief medical officer, Professor Dame Sally Davies, has said this may be the first generation of children that is outlived by its parents.

The rocketing levels of obesity and the diseases associated with it has left no socio-economic class, age or demographic immune across the western world. It's even affected the military. In 2012, the Surgeon General of the United States declared that obesity was now a threat to America's national security.

However, obesity itself is just the tip of an enormous iceberg of chronic diseases driven by poor lifestyle, namely, heart disease, type-2 diabetes, cancer and dementia. In the United States, 75 per cent of over 3 trillion healthcare dollars are now spent treating these diseases; and they also lie behind most of the demand on the UK's National Health Service.

And it's not just our health services that are struggling to cope with this avalanche of illness. An unhealthy, unhappy society is also an economically unproductive one.

How have we allowed this to happen? Is it down to lack of personal responsibility? Could gluttony and slothfulness be eliminated, or substantially reduced by the simple educational message: eat less and move more? No – this is not the case; in fact, this is one of several fatally flawed messages which, in addition to making us sicker has also detracted from the introduction of truly meaningful solutions both for individuals and for the wider population at large.

Be prepared for everything you know and believe to be true to be turned on its head. Misguided public health messages and the marketing campaigns that push them continue to mislead doctors, the public and politicians, but it's time for that to change.

The following chapters will explode several myths, including why you need to stop fearing saturated fat and cholesterol, why you must stop counting calories, why an ageing population is not really an issue and that you can drop dead healthy, why there's no such thing as a 'healthy weight', and why sugar deserves its reputation as public enemy number one in the western diet. Once you understand the science behind this, you will be better equipped to commence and experience what will be the beginning of a life-changing journey taking just twenty-one days.

The Pioppi Diet combines and layers multiple 'health positive' lifestyle choices – of which food is but one – to fire up your body's feel-good factor. While it is, generally speaking, the main determinant of health, the impact of better food choices will be magnified by making more informed choices in other areas of our daily habitual lifestyle. It is the combination of these factors that makes the Pioppi Diet uniquely powerful as a twenty-one-day health intervention. In simple terms, the Pioppi Diet is designed to help you tune into your body and recognize and respond to its requirements: food, sleep, movement, breathing and 'exercise' – which we prefer to call 'mindful movement'. The result is a subtle but incredibly powerful demonstration of your body's ability to lead you towards a leaner, healthier, happier and more energized you.

But don't just take our word for it. We are privileged to engage the expertise and support of a multitude of respected international scientists, including cardiologists and obesity experts. With this, combined with our own experience and other personal testimonials, you can feel confident that the solutions of the Pioppi Diet are driven by the best available modern scientific evidence. This book is based on the 2016 documentary film *The Big Fat Fix*, which was co-produced by me and former international athlete and film-maker Donal O'Neill. The former Secretary of State for Health and current Mayor of Greater Manchester, Andy Burnham, has publicly recognized the film's potential 'to help millions and save thousands of lives' – our ultimate and most important goal – and I would ask and actively encourage you to share the health secrets of the Pioppi Diet with family, friends and colleagues far and wide. Trust me, it is never too soon – or too late – to make positive lifestyle changes.

To quote a young editor of *Men's Health* magazine who transformed his health and life by adopting these changes, 'This stuff really works.'

PART ONE
The Story and the Science

1.

Pioppi:
The Village Where
People Forget to Die

'In Italy, in the Campania region, in the
province of Salerno, in Cilento, in Pollica,
we have a treasure.'

– Stefano Pisani, Mayor of Campania, June 2015,
in an interview for *The Big Fat Fix*

Never have truer words been spoken.

In southern Italy, two hours south of Naples, there is a tiny village called Pioppi (population: 197). Every day, a handful of small boats leaves the picture-book harbour to fish for their designated catch. The fishermen's bounty is more communal than commercial. The boats return with enough to sustain the community and the very small number of local restaurants. Each afternoon, all the people in this village (which doesn't have a supermarket) retire for the traditional siesta. Local legend has it that the character of Santiago in Ernest Hemingway's *Old Man and the Sea* (1952) was inspired by a visit by the author to the region. If you visit – as we did – you will find that very easy to believe.

After my father suffered a heart attack in 2010, I spent the following five years researching the ins and outs of heart disease and our modern diet. Not long before that heart attack, my dad had been congratulated when he sailed through his most recent cardiac stress test. 'Are you an athlete, Mr O'Neill?' he was asked. 'Not any more,' he replied. 'But I was a long time ago.'

Like many households, we had replaced butter with 'heart healthy' margarine back in the 1980s. In one TV advert, fat was poured down a kitchen sink to demonstrate the operation of saturated fat in clogging your arteries. Not only was this a devastatingly effective visual, it carried an equally compelling – though ultimately misleading – message. My mum began to cook with 'healthy' sunflower oil, and full-cream was replaced with semi-skimmed milk in our house. We all feared fat.

That narrative would stay with me until 2010, when my research for *Cereal Killers* began. When we eventually stumbled over the line with that movie in 2013, Aseem embraced the movie and its message. He organized screenings in London and invited key medical and media figures to attend, and my appearance on *BBC Breakfast* with Dr Peter Brukner, the former Head of Sports Medicine and Sports Science at Liverpool Football Club and now team doctor to the Australian cricket team, was entirely his doing.

'Don't Fear Fat' was the tagline to *Cereal Killers*. If it seemed an outrageous and rebellious message at the time (one national broadcaster was keen to commission a remake, 'only with much less fat'), public feeling has shifted in the interim. When we pointed the camera towards athletic performance and to the remarkable Sami Inkinen for our follow-up documentary, *Run on Fat*, there was no grand plan to make a third movie. But then I read about Pioppi in Nina Teicholz's excellent book *The Big Fat Surprise*, and I wondered if there was a story waiting to be told in this tiny, long-forgotten Italian village. When internet searches came up with nothing on the subject, I got very excited indeed.

It was June 2015 when we arrived, unannounced, in Pioppi to film *The Big Fat Fix*. The brief was to capture the very essence of a sleepy little village where the people forget to die. This proved to be straightforward on the one hand, but almost impossible on the other.

Where there was food, we would shoot it. When we enjoyed food, we would discuss it on camera. But in our bid to recover the true secrets of Mediterranean longevity, we were planning to go beyond food. Way beyond. As we opened our senses to invite the magic of this environment to seep into our bones, we came to identify and peel back those forgotten layers of lifestyle – the 'treasure' referred to by the mayor – which had been buried by decades of misinformation.

When I sat down to a seafood lunch on that first day with Aseem – by then my co-producer, co-author in waiting and leading global anti-obesity campaigner – I stopped thinking there might be a story and started to believe there might be much more than that. We both did.

The restaurant we chose to focus on was La Caupona, in the heart of the village, and the hospitality we enjoyed that afternoon set the tone for a remarkable stay in this magical place. We spoke no Italian, and the elderly gentleman who greeted, served and waved us goodbye spoke no English. His mode of communication was his enormous smile, but we nonetheless navigated our way to a remarkable feast of seafood, grilled vegetables and an abundance of olive oil.

As Aseem smoothly extolled the heart-healthy virtues of olive oil to the camera, Marek, the cameraman, salivated behind it. As a general rule, when the guy behind the camera is genuinely interested in what's happening in front of it, you're probably winning, so this was a good start. Like all good directors, our director, Yolanda, likes to plan shooting schedules carefully, but when nobody speaks English and you don't quite know what you're looking for in the first instance, sometimes you have to go with your gut. This is not how documentaries are typically made, of course, but it very often makes for a better film.

When Professor Tim Noakes referred to *The Big Fat Fix* as 'exceptional. The best health movie ever' and Aseem secured a worldwide premiere screening to members of the British Parliament in Westminster, we felt that we had successfully navigated our way to a solid end result. Of course, on our first day of filming, we had no idea that this was to come.

There was a lot we didn't know.

After lunch, we drove around to familiarize ourselves

with the area while the locals retired for their siesta. We would come to appreciate the potential – and very powerful – health significance of that cultural daily rite, but, like many of the lifestyle elements we identified in our time in Pioppi, it is impossible to isolate any one factor as an elixir of the remarkable health and longevity the people of this region have traditionally enjoyed.

When you read about the longevity research and 'findings' of those scientists who followed in our footsteps, we would urge you to take their recommendations of singularly magical longevity herbs with a pinch of sea salt. Our movie and this book recognize Pioppi as a very special place where impeccable traits of medical, nutritional and environmental science coexist, collide and combine with the physical wisdom of the very long-living in a perfect storm of human potential. The reality is simple enough. Science knows much less than we think and the people of Pioppi know a lot more than we have given them credit for – until now.

Pioppi is a place where time stretches, cradling you into a very compelling sense that not much matters beyond the minuscule borders of the village. The still and quiet of our first night there was a silent wrecking ball to our typical nocturnal environments. No noise. No lights. No disturbances of any kind at all. Just complete, idyllic serenity.

We woke the next day to a collective realization that our impromptu visit was becoming an immersion into something very special indeed. How to convert that into something tangible for the viewer was our next major hurdle. On that crisp, clear morning in southern Italy, it struck us that there was only one way to start that process.

Coffee.

The espresso bar in the centre of the village sits across the small open square from the restaurant where we had dined so well the day before. We successfully sign-languaged our way to espressos, cappuccinos and, in keeping with the plan, filmed the process. The science behind coffee as a health-positive habitual drink is increasingly compelling, so we needed some 'cutaway' visuals to back this up in the movie. If the coffee itself was magnificent, there was a much more powerful message awakening in each of us that morning.

Scientists don't like to use the word 'stress' because it is not something they can accurately measure (the closest useable proxy is heart-rate variability (HRV), which we will discuss in more detail later). Although it is a very loose, catch-all term, 'stress' is something we each have an innate understanding of. We intuitively know when we ourselves, a family member, close friend or partner might be stressed and, over time, the implications of this on health can be profoundly deleterious.

The gut can respond very adversely to an increase in stress hormones, becoming more porous and effectively opening the door to invite illness in. While some experts in the field firmly believe that chronic stress is more damaging than even poor dietary choices in the long term, the one thing everyone agrees on is that less is much, much more when it comes to stress – pretty impressive for something we can't even 'measure' accurately.

Within twenty-four hours of arriving in Pioppi, as Aseem and I enjoyed looking out to sea while sipping our espressos, bathing in morning sunshine and pondering the treasure beneath our feet, we agreed that there was something intangible but very powerful in the air. The complete absence of stress as we perceive and experience it in a modern, urban environment was as clear as our view of pollution-free sea softly lapping the pristine pebbled beach below us. Pioppi may lie in a historically poor region of Italy, but its health bounty is rich, plentiful and unadulterated.

No gym. No supermarket. No problem.

In the 1970s, decades before the internet would suggest it might be possible, would it have been conceivable that this tiny village could assert a greater influence on global nutritional and health policies than anywhere else on the planet? The fact that it did just that is what brought Aseem and me to this remarkable place that morning. We were retracing the footsteps of the American scientist Professor Ancel Keys.

When he visited the region after the Second World War (he had, famously, invented the K-ration, a portable, non-perishable ration containing enough calories to sustain a soldier for up to two weeks), Keys was so taken with Pioppi that he would return years later, to conduct the research that has ultimately framed our modern, albeit skewed, interpretation of the traditional Mediterranean lifestyle. As the architect of the modern 'Mediterranean Diet', Keys and his wife, Margaret, would live and work among the people of Pioppi for four decades before his death in 2004. His name is still spoken with reverence and no short measure of affection there.

Road signs as you enter Pioppi from either side paying homage to Keys and the village's UNESCO-acknowledged status as the home of the Mediterranean Diet assured us that we were on the right trail. The official Mediterranean Diet Museum in an historic old building in the centre of the village satisfied us entirely that we had found the source of the greatest diet ever sold.

Pioppi booms in August as a destination for Italian holiday-makers but positively slumbers outside that small, blisteringly hot window. In the month of June, we figured the population of 197 would have immediately noticed the appearance of a camera crew in their midst. All we needed now was a means of communication more audible than the chorus of smiles which greeted us everywhere. Yolanda always says that a camera in public brings a sprinkle of magic with it. You never know who or what might present itself.

Angelo Morinelli was enjoying his morning espresso when a six-foot-five-inch cameraman appeared over his shoulder to capture the barista and the crema in close-up. He did not know that the man outside enjoying an espresso was Aseem Malhotra, a British cardiologist heading up a global campaign for lifestyle medicine. He would not have seen *Cereal Killers* either, but he knew enough to know that something was happening here.

And that he could probably help.

With no common language at our disposal, Marek's pidgin German saved the day, and he formally introduced us to the man who had been Ancel Keys's personal driver. It transpired that Angelo's father had owned the land where Keys would build his villa and, later, the complex he used to accommodate visiting scientists – Minnelea.

Angelo excitedly made a call and passed the phone to me. His son, Antonio, had recently returned home to Pioppi after a decade cooking in the US. As an ambitious young chef, he had been determined to open a top-quality restaurant in his home village. That was the dream: a tribute to local produce in the UNESCO-protected home of the Mediterranean Diet.

For the remainder of our time in Pioppi, Antonio would become our guide, our host and our friend. That evening, we ate in his restaurant, Suscettibile, for the first time. His dream had become a splendid reality. The fact that Suscettibile would excel anywhere in the world will surprise no one who has had the opportunity to dine there. There is love of place and produce and artistry on every plate. The buffalo mozzarella from the region is sublime, the seafood incomparable and the wine – ah, the wine!

That was the night we met the magnificent 'meditation' red. Antonio encouraged us to do so and then scheduled a visit to the magnificent San Giovanni winery to appreciate this local Mediterranean marvel. To see vines dive perilously down towards the sea with Pompei imperious in the distance sounds as improbable as it, in truth, appeared to the naked eye. If the camera struggled to capture the surreal beauty of this place, the wine did not. Ida Budetta explained how she and her husband had initially tilled this small plot of land with their bare hands. The term 'organic' means nothing here. There is just the land. And the sea. And the people's love of what they do. If the relationship with the land and its produce is one of mutual respect, this reflects a critical, forgotten aspect of the traditional lifestyle in this region – the work.

Antonio also arranged, and joined us for, our interview with Mayor Pisani. In one brief soundbite, the mayor explained in very simple terms where it had all gone wrong in the modern interpretation of the Mediterranean 'diet'. In a catastrophic case of 'lost in translation', the original greek word *diaita* had been misunderstood at its source. *Diaita* means 'lifestyle', and 'within that,' Pisani said, 'we include many things – the landscape, the sea, quality of life, culture, the work and many other things.'

In this region, the men, who work for eight hours a day, every day, in the fields, their entire adult life, outlive the local women. They outlive their peers around the world by almost a decade. These men joked with us about the intensity of chopping wood; it is part and parcel of their daily tasks. 'Try it for an hour,' they said, laughing. The 'work' the mayor referred to meant decades of slow, constant, habitual movement (walking) along with more intense, strength-maintaining bursts of full-body activity (wood chopping, and so on). Could it be a contributing factor to their longevity?

As we sought to marry the latest scientific research with the wisdom of this place and these people, the importance of movement and mobility became apparent. If the research aligning mobility with ten-year mortality rates (death from any cause) points to the importance of strength, balance and power as we age, the men of Pioppi need not worry.

The fact that science measures only that which it can – and, typically, only at acute points in time – and that modern medicine is essentially the business of illness management has created a vacuum in our understanding of how to truly live well. Healthy people do not interface with modern medicine in the same way as sick folks, if at all. While vast resources are ploughed into understanding, diagnosing and treating illnesses, the healthy are left alone to get on with living without illness. However, all bets are off when they reach a hundred or achieve some remarkable feat, at which point everyone suddenly wonders what they did to get there in the first place!

The power of myriad health-positive lifestyle choices (conscious or otherwise) such as those contained in a traditional lifestyle in Pioppi goes unnoticed until longer-term population trends emerge. Science then scurries to understand retrospectively how these people are consistently winning the longevity Olympics.

And they do not just live long, they live well.

If ageing is seen as a process of gradual physical deterioration, then the traditional people of Pioppi clearly accumulate the slings and arrows of that process more slowly than many of us. For example, it did not strike us as at all odd when we noticed our waiter from that first day helping to fix the roof of his premises one morning. When Antonio later informed us that he was eighty-five years old, we decided it was damned impressive. That his movements were fluid and trouble free certainly belied his chronological age. Unfortunately, our enthusiastic bubble was quickly burst when he then told us about another Antonio, the oldest man in the area, having reached the ripe old age of 107! While eighty-five might be considered an excellent innings anywhere else, our waiter was but a spring chicken in this village where the people forget to die.

So how exactly do they do it? The truth is, we will never be able to explain fully why these people live so well for so long, but we can certainly present the case for some authoritative guiding principles.

During an excellent tour of the Mediterranean Diet Museum in Pioppi with local English-language teacher Susan Bessie Haslam, it was pointed out to us that poverty would have exercised a strong impact on the traditional way of life in this region. Day to day, that meant restrictions on the availability of food and imposed windows of restricted eating. In this context, Antonio explained how the men would have gone to work the fields on an empty stomach on such occasions. Of course, we now know that fasting is a rising star in the treatment of type-2 diabetes and that bodybuilders have been using intermittent fasting protocols as a mechanism to manipulate lean muscle mass for some time now. It may not have been intentional, but intermittent fasting was a natural part of a traditional life in this region.

Although Ancel Keys's original research never accounted for periods of fasting or abstinence for religious or other reasons, it was a very real phenomenon across the Mediterranean after the Second World War. Just as the work would have contributed to the health benefits of the traditional *diaita*, so, too, the intermittent absence of food would have bestowed further marginal but meaningful gains for population health in the region. More on that later.

Like in a cryptic crossword, the clues to longevity were slowly presenting themselves everywhere we turned.

With hindsight, one can now see how the case for a super-simple interpretation of a much broader, potently health-positive lifestyle gathered momentum and credibility, first with Keys's researchers and, subsequently, with those policy-makers in the US who butchered the *diaita* through the prism of food politics in the 1970s.

The Pioppi Diet is a translation of what the governing lifestyle principles of a traditional Mediterranean *diaita* might look like in the context of a modern western lifestyle. Whether you are in New York, London or Sydney, we trust you will enjoy your own journey to better cardiovascular, physical and mental health and longevity.

In the chapters ahead, you will learn more about the root cause of modern lifestyle diseases, including heart disease, obesity and type-2 diabetes. We will explain why exercise has been overrated – and movement underrated – as a weight-loss mechanism; what telomeres are and why effective stress management is a critically important tool to protect them; which foods can radically impact on your body composition, energy levels and cardiovascular health. Most importantly, you will be given a clear set of guidelines and an easy-to-follow, Pioppi-influenced prescription for better health that will dramatically reduce your risk of heart disease in just twenty-one days.

If you can't wait to get started on that plan, you can jump right ahead to Chapter 14. A word of warning, though! When your family, friends and colleagues ask why you're looking and feeling so good in three weeks' time, you may have to circle back to understand what exactly just happened. Then again, you could just tell them, 'It's all about Pioppi.'

If the future of healthcare is lifestyle medicine, then Pioppi was way ahead of its time!

2.

The Pioppi Diet: A Healthcare Manifesto

'Let food be thy medicine, and medicine be thy food.'

– Hippocrates (the father of modern medicine)

I don't believe anyone chooses to be overweight. A 2013 Gallup international survey of 57,000 adults revealed that it is health that matters most in life, followed by a happy family environment. But how can this be reconciled with the fact that 60 per cent of adults in the UK are currently overweight or obese and, perhaps of greater concern, that one in three children are in the same category by the time they leave primary school? And things are set to get worse, not better.

There are two fundamental misunderstandings among the scientific community and the public that continue to inhibit attempts to solve this epidemic. The first is our collective and individual failure to recognize that what we put in our mouths every time we eat can either confer wellness or contribute to a ticking bomb of chronic disease and early death. This is not just a philosophical construct. As the diagram below shows, poor diet now contributes more to disease and death globally than does lack of physical activity, smoking and alcohol combined.

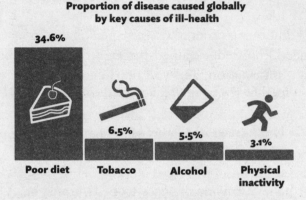

Proportion of disease caused globally by key causes of ill-health

34.6% Poor diet

6.5% Tobacco

5.5% Alcohol

3.1% Physical inactivity

Source: Prof Simon Capewell, Professor of Clinical Epidemiology, University of Liverpool, analysis of Lancet global burden of disease report

Credit: Simon Capewell and the *Telegraph*

In 2017, it was estimated that a collective improvement in diet in the US could save $1.8 trillion of the current $3.2 trillion spent on healthcare.[1]

The second misconception is the belief that our food choices are made deliberately and reflect our true desires, when the reality is that the decisions we make about what we eat are often difficult to control and made without full conscious awareness. As Professor Theresa Marteau, Director of the Behaviour and Health Research Unit at the University of Cambridge, says, 'We are heavily influenced by automatic behaviours which require little cognition, where the desire for instant gratification far outweighs greater, less assured and more distant rewards to make us more likely to act in unhealthy ways.' Despite wishing to lose weight, for example, we're still tempted to buy the brightly coloured chocolate bar at the check-out in the supermarket.

In addition, in order to exercise personal responsibility, you need knowledge gained through the assimilation of correct information, and you need choice. We have neither. A combination of flawed dietary advice, combined with a food environment that inhibits our ability to make healthy choices, means that, for most people, personal responsibility is nothing more than an illusion. Navigating our way through the oversupply of cheap, processed foods blitzed by aggressive marketing for junk food by an industry whose 'low fat', 'gluten free' or 'heart healthy' health claims are more likely to damage your health is not easy. Take, for instance, a patient of mine in her forties, who, after suffering a heart attack, primarily brought on by years of heavy smoking, couldn't understand why she'd gained three stone in weight after adopting a 'low fat' diet. She was horrified when I pointed out that the five low-fat milk drinks she was getting through daily contained a total of seventy-five teaspoons of sugar. I now tell my patients to avoid buying anything that's marketed as 'healthy', as it's likely to have the opposite impact on your health.

However, I don't blame the food industry entirely. Their obligation is to make a profit from selling food, not to look after consumers' health. It's in curbing their excesses and manipulations that we have failed. Leading researcher on public policy in the US Professor Kelly Brownell said, 'When the history of the world's attempt to address obesity is written, one of the greatest failures may be collaboration with and appeasement of the food industry.'[2] The industry has managed to make their nutritionally poor yet highly palatable junk food and drink available to anyone, anywhere, any time.

For me personally, and as a doctor, the biggest scandal is that we've even allowed our hospitals to become a branding opportunity for the junk-food industry. After performing a life-saving procedure on a middle-aged man suffering a heart attack in the middle of the night a number of years ago, I still vividly recall his words on the ward round the next day. As I was counselling him on the importance of stopping smoking and of a healthy diet (most of his weekly diet consisted of fast food), he was served up a burger and chips by the healthcare assistant. He looked at me and said, 'How do you expect me to change my lifestyle if you're serving me the same crap that brought me here in the first place?'

The fact that 50 per cent of the 1.4 million people working in the National Health Service are overweight or obese is a clear indication that education is ineffective when the food environment around you is working against you.[3]

Eating and living more healthily is not just about delaying death. It is about having a healthier and happier quality of life now *and* in our later years. Remember that sprightly

85-year-old man in Pioppi? Both Donal and I hope that we are as agile and as mentally sharp as he is when we get to his age. And, given a choice, I'd rather drop dead healthy than live the last decade of my life with a disability I could have avoided.

'Ageing population' is a term we are hearing cited more and more as a cause of the increase in demand on our health services. But although a population may be ageing, demands for healthcare will increase substantially only if those later years are accompanied by chronic disease. An analysis published in the *Lancet* found that, if rising life expectancy in the European Union was characterized by years of good health, health expenditure on an ageing population would be expected to increase by only 0.7 per cent of Gross Domestic Product (GDP) by 2060.[4]

In other words, it's having an ageing population with chronic disease driven predominantly by lifestyle factors that's the major issue. And, added to this, there's the economic toll of the increase in prevalence of type-2 diabetes affecting younger and younger adults. The combined cost of type-2 diabetes to the NHS and lost productivity due to sickness from work is currently close to £20 billion; if we continue as we are, this will double to £40 billion in less than twenty years.[5]

A report by investment bank Morgan Stanley has predicted that, unless drastic action is taken, the 'diabesity' epidemic will result in 0.0 per cent economic growth in the US by 2035. They conclude, 'If the diabesity trend starts to slow, stop – even reverse – the effects could be startling.

Imagine healthier communities; more productive working populations; less financial drag on individual, corporate and government budgets; stronger economic growth at a global scale.'[6]

And improving health and quality of life is certainly not going to happen from more mass pill-popping. Because of side effects, it has been estimated that prescription medications are now the third most common cause of death globally, after heart disease and cancer. It's estimated that up to a quarter of hospital admissions in the elderly are a result of dangerous drug interactions. The side effects of blood-pressure pills, for example, can result in falls. And a quarter of elderly patients who fall and break a hip will subsequently die in hospital after admission.

So why are we all living longer?

Although there is no doubt that modern medicine has accomplished some remarkable things in the last century, such as the discovery of antibiotics to treat life-threatening infections and emergency key-hole surgery for heart attacks, twenty-five of the thirty-year average increase in life expectancy in the US since 1900 has occurred through government regulation. This includes compulsory seat belts in cars, better sanitation, safer work environments, safe drinking water and smoke-free buildings.

In fact, as I'll explain in more detail later, the reduction in the prevalence of smoking over the past thirty years has been the single most important factor driving the reduction in death rates from heart disease in the population.

And this has occurred only through public-health interventions and campaigns that specifically targeted the availability, affordability and acceptability of tobacco. Many of my patients who have suffered heart attacks have been nudged to give up smoking because the price of cigarettes has gone up.

Oxford University researchers have calculated that a 20 per cent tax on sugary drinks will prevent 180,000 people from becoming obese and over 200,000 from becoming overweight within a year.[7]

The UK will be introducing a tax on sugary drinks from April 2018, following in the footsteps of France, Finland, Hungary and Mexico. Mexico has seen average decline of almost 8 per cent in the consumption of such beverages within two years of introducing a sugary-drinks tax of 10 per cent. It's been estimated that this could prevent almost 200,000 new cases of type-2 diabetes, 20,400 strokes and heart attacks and 18,900 deaths among adults aged between thirty-five and ninety-four between 2013 and 2022. Just reducing the burden of type-2 diabetes alone could save Mexico almost $1 billion; almost 70 per cent of the population are currently overweight or obese.

As the Center of Disease Control health impact pyramid below shows, making the default food choice the healthy choice will have significantly more impact on population health than individual counselling or education. It's like telling a child who grows up in a sweet shop not to eat sweets.[8]

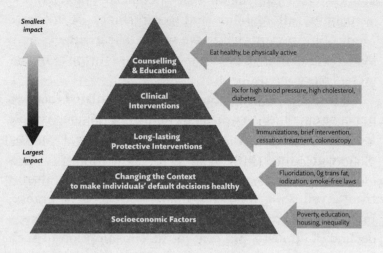

Smallest impact

Largest impact

Counselling & Education — Eat healthy, be physically active

Clinical Interventions — Rx for high blood pressure, high cholesterol, diabetes

Long-lasting Protective Interventions — Immunizations, brief intervention, cessation treatment, colonoscopy

Changing the Context to make individuals' default decisions healthy — Fluoridation, 0g trans fat, iodization, smoke-free laws

Socioeconomic Factors — Poverty, education, housing, inequality

The sustainability of the Pioppi Diet in the longer term will be helped by a collective effort to make our food environment healthier so that you, and all those you interact with, whether it be loved ones, friends or work colleagues, can ultimately swim with the current, not against the tide.

In order for this to happen, medical training must adapt and change. It may come as a surprise to you, but the overwhelming majority of doctors are not equipped with even basic training to give specific, evidence-based lifestyle advice to individuals. I don't remember receiving a single lecture at medical school on the impact of nutrition and lifestyle on preventing and treating disease.

Only from my own research, and many years after qualifying as a medical doctor, have I concluded that adopting a high-fat Mediterranean diet, quitting smoking and engaging in mindful movement and stress reduction are more powerful than any drug in the prevention and treatment of many chronic diseases, including heart disease.

Last year, I and a number of prominent doctors, sports scientists and nutritionists wrote a widely publicized letter to the General Medical Council (GMC) and Medical School's Council (MSC) calling for the compulsory introduction of evidence-based lifestyle education into all medical curricula.

A global survey carried out by investment bank Credit Suisse reveals, worryingly, a substantial level of misinformation existing among doctors, with 92 per cent believing that fat consumption could lead to cardiovascular issues. Fifty-four per cent of doctors and 40 per cent of nutritionists incorrectly thought that eating cholesterol-rich foods raises blood cholesterol.[9]

A survey of medical students carried out by the Physical Activity Research Unit in Edinburgh revealed that only 14.9 per cent knew what the Chief Medical Officer's physical activity guidelines were, and only 10 per cent felt adequately trained to give advice on physical activity. However, the good news is that 90 per cent of these students wanted more formal training in this area.[10]

Another heartening survey, this time by New York University, revealed that, when it comes to nutrition, 78 per cent of physicians were willing to undergo further training because they believed it would benefit patients.[11]

Towards the end of his life, the pioneering heart-transplant surgeon Christiaan Barnard said, with some regret, 'I have saved the lives of 150 people through heart transplants. If I had concentrated on preventative medicine earlier, I could have saved 150 million.' As it turns out, lifestyle, the Pioppi Diet, is that medicine.

In summary:

- Health tops the list of what's most important to people in life

- Globally poor diet is responsible for more disease and death than lack of physical activity, smoking and alcohol combined

- Prescription medications are the third most common cause of death after heart disease and cancer

- A healthy ageing population is not a threat to the health service or to the economy

- Making healthy food the default choice through regulation will have more impact on population health than individual counselling or education

3.
What is Processed Food?

The following are the nutritional properties and markers that distinguish processed food, as laid down by one of the leading voices on child obesity in the US, Professor Robert Lustig, in an article in *JAMA Pediatrics* of January 2017. (Sections in italics are additions by the authors.)

1. **Too little fibre.** When fibre is eaten with food, it forms a barrier along the intestinal wall which delays the speed of absorption of glucose, while simultaneously feeding the gut microbiome (see p. 70). This reduction in the rapid rise of glucose reduces insulin secretion. Fibre also decreases fructose absorption, which attenuates liver-fat build-up. You may think your liver isn't damaged by a gentle tap of fructose, but it will be if it receives several punches. Thus: eat the fruit, *don't* drink the juice (see Chapter 4).

2. **Too few omega-3 and too many omega-6 fatty acids.** Omega-3s are precursors of docosahexaenoic acid and eicosapentaenoic acids (anti-inflammatory), but omega-6 fatty acids are

precursors of arachidonic acid (proinflammatory). Our blood-ratio levels of omega 6 to omega 3 should be at least 1:3, and closer to 1:1, but current ratios are actually closer to 25:1, inducing a pro-inflammatory state, which can drive oxidative stress and cell damage (see Chapter 7; specifically, why you should avoid cooking in seed oils).

3. **Too few micronutrients.** Vitamin C and vitamin E are antioxidants and help prevent cell damage. Other micronutrients, such as carotenoids, help reduce lipid peroxidation; in other words, they reduce cholesterol's ability to damage arteries.

   Foods high in vitamin E include almonds, spinach, sweet potato and avocado. Foods high in vitamin C include bell peppers, green chillies, dark leafy greens broccoli, berries, citrus fruits and tomatoes.

   Carotenoids are vitamin-like pigments contained within many fruits and vegetables. High quantities are found in foods such as sweet potato, green leafy vegetables and tomatoes.

4. **Too many trans fats.** Trans fats have traditionally been a common constituent of packaged, boxed food and fast food, especially if it is deep-fried. In 2013, the US Food and Drug Administration (FDA) removed it from a list of foods 'generally recognized as safe' so, hopefully,

it will soon disappear from the food supply. Over the years, the decline in its consumption has been one major factor in the reduction in death rates from heart disease.

5. **Too many branched-chain amino acids.** Valine, leucine and isoleucine are essential amino acids needed for muscle biosynthesis and are found in foods such as meat and eggs. However, if they are consumed in excess, they will be converted to liver fat and increase the risk of insulin resistance.

6. **Too many emulsifiers.** Emulsifiers keep fat and water in food such as ice cream or lasagne from separating. However, they are detergents and may strip away the mucin layer that protects intestinal epithelial cells and hence contribute to a predisposition to intestinal disease or food allergy.

7. **Too many nitrates.** Nitrates (processed meat) can be metabolized into nitrosoureas, which have been linked to colon cancer.

8. **Excessive salt.** About 15 per cent of the population is salt sensitive, and in those with high blood pressure, in particular, excessive salt can increase the risk of heart attack, stroke and heart failure.

9. **Too much alcohol.** Excess alcohol is converted to liver fat and drives insulin resistance and metabolic syndrome (a cluster of risk factors that includes type-2 diabetes, high blood pressure, increased waist circumference, high triglycerides and low HDL cholesterol). Small doses of red wine have been shown to be protective against the development of heart disease, as long as you keep within the recommended maximum limit of fourteen units a week (one glass of red wine a day), you'll be just fine!

10. **Too much fructose.** Excessive fructose, most commonly ingested in the form of sucrose or high-fructose corn syrup, is linked to an adverse cholesterol profile that increases the risk of heart disease, type-2 diabetes, fatty-liver disease, high blood pressure (through its effects on uric acid), cancer and, last but not least, obesity.

4.

Why Pick On Sugar?

'Sugar is the only substance that humans ingest
that has no nutritional value whatsoever, no
essential fats, no protein, no vitamins, no
minerals . . . in terms of sugar, we either eat it on
top of what we should be eating, in which case it
can make us fat, or we eat it instead of what we
should be eating, which leaves us nutritionally
deficient and we end up sick. So we're getting fat
and sick at the same time.'

– Dr Zoe Harcombe, PhD, Public Health
Nutrition Researcher

Actually, there is one other substance that meets these
criteria: alcohol. Alcohol is not a nutrient either, and alcohol and sugar bear striking similarities in the ways in
which they work on your liver and your brain.

But Dr Harcombe is absolutely correct, of course. Contrary to what the food industry may wish you to believe, the
human body has no biological requirement for added sugar
whatsoever, and sugar is therefore not a 'nutrient' and

should be described only as an ingredient or additive. When we refer to 'added sugar', we are discussing sucrose (50 per cent glucose and 50 per cent fructose) or high-fructose corn syrup (45 per cent glucose and 55 per cent fructose).

As a consequence of this, many describe added sugar simply as empty calories – but the scientific evidence paints a much bleaker picture when it comes to our health.

Firstly, when it comes to teeth, sugar is one of the only substances we ingest that is directly corrosive to teeth enamel. In the UK, tooth decay is not only the main cause of chronic pain but is the number-one driver of admissions to hospital among young children. And tooth decay is a significant problem for adults, too. In industrialized countries between 5 and 10 per cent of GDP is spent treating dental disease which is almost entirely avoidable. To put this in perspective, in parts of Nigeria, which has almost no consumption of sugar (approximately half a teaspoon a day), only 2 per cent of the population has tooth decay, whereas in the US almost 92 per cent of the population has suffered from tooth decay in at least one of their permanent teeth.[1]

There are now eighty-seven studies on the adverse effects of added sugar on health (and not a single one showing any benefits).[2] We will look at a few of these to explain why everyone, no matter what shape or size, is vulnerable to the harms of excess sugar.

However, before we do, let's briefly summarize the biological mechanism whereby sugar directly and indirectly harms the body (in addition to its negative impact on teeth). Glucose is a molecule that is necessary for life: it's used by every cell and directly enters the bloodstream from the stomach, any excess being stored in the liver as glycogen, to be used at a later stage when needed. Yet even glucose in excess, and in volume and concentration, has a detrimental effect on health: it drives the pancreas to release more insulin, and therefore more energy deposits, into fat tissue, and therefore contributes to weight gain. However, it's the fructose component of sugar that is uniquely deleterious. Rather like alcohol, fructose is not essential to life and is almost entirely metabolized by the liver because it cannot be directly converted into energy by other organs. Paediatric endocrinologist Professor Robert Lustig describes fructose as the 'alcohol of the child', and he's right. When consumed in excess, it promotes a process known as de novo lipogenesis. In other words, it gets converted to fat, some of which causes the liver to build up fat, which promotes hepatic insulin resistance (discussed later), and some of which is released as triglycerides into the bloodstream, affecting a person's cholesterol profile adversely (see Chapter 6). Another thing fructose does is to generate excessive reactive oxygen species which directly damage our cells, promoting their dysfunction and death and inducing the production of inflammatory cytokines. Reactive oxygen species are directly implicated in the development of cardiovascular disease and cancer.

Fructose also interferes with hormones that control appetite and, as a result, one is not only left not feeling full but, as many people, including myself, often experience, you become hungry again in a much shorter time period. I tell my patients when encouraging them to cut out sugar – or, at the very least, to drastically reduce the amount of sugar they're consuming – to treat sugar as an appetite stimulant.

Beyond obesity (calculated by body mass index (BMI)), chronic exposure to fructose has a direct effect on promoting the accumulation of liver fat, insulin resistance and metabolic syndrome. And metabolic syndrome and its precursor, insulin resistance (see Chapter 7), are in fact bigger problems than obesity, because up to 40 per cent of people of 'normal' weight will harbour metabolic abnormalities which those with obesity have as a result of lifestyle factors. These include cardiovascular disease, high blood pressure, type-2 diabetes and fatty-liver disease. Conversely, 20 per cent of those classified as obese will be metabolically normal.[3] Think rugby players! In other words, two people with exactly the same BMI can have polar opposite markers of metabolic health. Therefore, there's no such thing as a 'healthy weight', only a healthy person!

Two of the most up-to-date and highest-quality landmark studies published in the past few years reveal that the negative effects of excess sugar consumption extend beyond just unnecessary calories. In 2013, researchers from Stanford University and the University of California, San Francisco, set out to determine what in the food environment predicted the increase in type-2 diabetes in the population. Looking at 175 countries across the world, they found that, for every excess 150 calories of sugar (typical of a can of cola) available for consumption, compared to 150 calories from fat or protein, there was an eleven-fold increase in the prevalence of type-2 diabetes, independent of body weight and levels of physical activity.[4]

In other words, even if you have a normal body mass index and exercise regularly, consuming too much sugar is associated with significantly increasing your risk of developing type-2 diabetes.

Another study, published in *JAMA Internal Medicine* in 2014, looked specifically at sugar consumption in the US population and found that those who consumed more than 25 per cent of their daily calories from sugar were three times more likely to die from cardiovascular disease than those who consumed less than 10 per cent of their calories from sugar. Yet again, these findings showed that these adverse effects were independent of weight and levels of physical activity.[5]

So how quickly can a reduction in sugar intake start to improve health markers? A recent study of forty-three African American and Latino children who had metabolic syndrome revealed that just nine days of cutting sugar from 28 per cent of calories consumed to less than 10 per cent had a significant impact on reducing triglycerides, LDL cholesterol, blood pressure and fasting insulin levels (total calories consumed from carbohydrate remained the same).[6]

Be aware that much of this added sugar is considered hidden; the majority of foods in the UK and 74 per cent of foods in US supermarkets contain added sugar, and much of it is not obvious. In the US, a third of sugar consumption comes from sugary drinks, a sixth from foods which one would normally characterize as junk foods, such as chocolate bars, cakes and biscuits, but almost half comes from food people wouldn't normally think of as having sugar in them, such as ketchup, salad dressings, cooking sauces and even bread.

We believe that people should exercise personal responsibility, but for that you need knowledge or information presented in an easy-to-understand manner and you need choice; and with misleading health claims on 'low fat' options that are in reality loaded with sugar, combined with sugar being almost unavoidable, it makes it difficult to choose healthy options.

To reiterate, although we hope you are now better armed to understand the science around sugar, we must also ensure that we create a food environment that makes it easier for us to make healthy choices. This means ensuring that the food industry stops spiking our food with added sugar and makes labelling easier for people to understand, by using teaspoons as a measure, for example, instead of what currently exists in the small print of nutritional information on foods such as 'carbohydrates, of which sugars . . .' Until that day comes, a relatively simple way is to divide the number of grams of sugar on the label by four. So four grams of sugar is approximately one teaspoon.

So, what is the optimum level of consumption? For the purposes of health, you guessed it. It's *zero*. But in small doses, sugar is unlikely to do harm and can be enjoyed. The World Health Organization (WHO) has now set a maximum-limit target per day for the average adult of no more than six teaspoons of added sugar or free sugar found in fruit juice, syrups and honey. The US Department of

Agriculture (USDA) recommends a maximum limit of no more than three teaspoons for children between four and eight years of age. Just to put it in perspective, one regular-sized chocolate bar, a glass of fruit juice or a can of cola contains at least twice and almost three times that amount! And the stark reality is that most of us in the UK and USA are consuming at least five to seven times the upper limit recommended by researchers at the London School of Tropical Medicine and Hygiene, and at least two to three times the maximum limit recommended by the World Health Organization.

In Pioppi, sugar was traditionally considered a rare treat. Sugar is synonymous with dessert, and how often would the people there traditionally eat dessert? Only on Sundays! But many people are effectively eating dessert two to three times a day. If you're having cereal for breakfast, a mid-morning biscuit, chocolate bar or fruit smoothie, and a slice of cake after dinner, you can see how this adds up. I myself used to be that person – on reflection, I was probably consuming forty teaspoons of sugar a day on occasion, and I thought that always being hungry was the norm until I started to research sugar myself. Now, other than the occasional treat, I do not consume any sugar as part of my regular healthy diet. My cholesterol profile is better than it's ever been and, by reducing my consumption of sugar and other refined carbohydrates, the fatty tyre around my waist has disappeared – something I thought I could never shift, despite pounding out five kilometres at the gym three times a week and lifting weights on the days in between.

As part of the Twenty-one-day Plan, we encourage you to go completely cold turkey – have *no* added sugar for the first two weeks, and then you can re-introduce it, if you wish, in small amounts, in the form of a square of dark chocolate (at least 85 per cent cocoa solids). In two weeks, you will experience what it feels like to be sugar free, break the addiction of sugar cravings (which may have become the norm in your life), and your taste buds, which have been desensitized from years of regular excess sugar consumption, will readjust.

In summary:

- The body has no biological requirement for added sugar

- The adverse effect of excess sugar consumption on health is independent of body weight or levels of physical activity

- The fructose component of added sugar interferes with the hormones that control appetite

- The World Health Organization recommends a maximum daily limit of added-sugar consumption of no more than six teaspoons a day; this includes fruit juice, syrups and honey

- Significantly cutting your intake of sugar can have a positive health impact within days

5.

Saturated Fat Does Not Clog the Arteries

'A retrospective cohort analysis of the Seven Countries Study revealed the food that correlated most with coronary mortality was sweets, not saturated fat from meat.'

– Nina Teicholz, investigative science journalist and author of *The Big Fat Surprise*

There can be no doubt he found treasure in Pioppi, but it now appears he buried some before he left. If Pioppi feels like a place you want to keep to yourself, one wonders if Keys was suitably motivated to do likewise with some of his own findings. For decades, the conventional wisdom has been that saturated fat from foods such as meat, butter, eggs and cheese clogs the arteries and so leads to heart attacks. This misconception arose from Keys's landmark Seven Countries Study, in which the American scientist demonstrated a correlation between the consumption of saturated fat in the diet and blood cholesterol levels and heart disease. Did the fact that he received funding from the sugar industry influence his decision to ignore its significance in the context of habitual consumption – or, specifically, lack thereof – across the Mediterranean region? And it was Keys's work in this study that led to a change in dietary advice in the US and UK in 1977 and 1983, respectively, to reduce total fat consumption to less than 30 per cent of calories consumed and, more specifically, saturated fat to less than 10 per cent of calories consumed. This is advice that I and many others now argue has in fact driven the twin epidemics of type-2 diabetes and obesity by increasing consumption of sugar, other refined carbohydrates and processed vegetable oils. A very well-researched report by Credit Suisse published in 2015 revealed that 90 per cent of the increase in calories in the American diet between 1961 and 2011 has come from refined carbohydrates and vegetable oils.[1] But from what we now understand of the biology around the development of heart disease, combined with robust modern scientific data, saturated fat in your diet does not clog the arteries, and it's just plain wrong to say that it does.

Before we get into the principle scientific studies addressing the question of the link between fat and saturated fat and heart disease, let's address some key facts and misconceptions, so you can come to understand that eating foods high in fat and saturated fat can instead be an important part of a healthy diet.

1. Fat in unprocessed food is a crucial provider of essential fats (linoleic acid and alpha-linolenic

acid) which are vital for immune function and to maintain the integrity of cells. Dietary fat is also essential in order for the body to obtain and absorb the fat-soluble vitamins A, D, E and K.

2. All unprocessed natural foods that are high in fat – meat, fish, eggs and dairy – contain saturated fat, just to differing degrees, together with unsaturated and polyunsaturated fat. Dairy foods are the only food group that contain more saturated than unsaturated fat. Even extra virgin olive oil, with varieties containing anything from 14 to 20 per cent saturated fat, contains many times more than the percentage of saturated fat in a pork chop.

3. Dietary fat is satiating. In other words, it helps you feel full for longer in comparison to refined carbohydrates and sugar and can therefore help you to control your weight.

4. In comparison to protein and carbohydrates, dietary fat has the least impact on raising blood glucose and thus spiking insulin. And it is insulin resistance that is the most important risk factor for heart attacks (see Chapter 7).

5. Some foods high in fat – in particular, extra virgin olive oil and nuts – have been proven to prevent heart attacks and strokes.

When Keys conducted the Seven Countries Study, many of the foods that were singled out as being high in saturated fat and harmful in their correlation with heart disease were processed carbohydrate foods such as cakes, ice cream, biscuits and pastries.[2]

This misconception is still propagated in the media. How many times have you seen articles or news stories on obesity in which eating fat or saturated fat are singled out as culprits and accompanied by a picture of an overweight person digging into a burger and fries? In fact, a typical beef burger (without the refined carbohydrate bun) has a total fat percentage of approximately 20 per cent, and sirloin steak has a saturated fat percentage of 2.1 per cent, well under the current recommended limit of 10 per cent a day.

The bun and chips is almost entirely refined carbohydrate, and is made even less healthy because the chips are cooked in vegetable oil (see Chapter 7).

Rather than call it fatty food, it would be far more accurate to describe burger and chips (a meal which almost everyone recognizes as junk food) as being made up predominantly of refined carbohydrates and vegetable oil. 'Fattening food' would be a much better description!

As a result of public-health messaging that has wrongly singled out fat and, in particular, saturated fat as being harmful, the food industry produced a market for supermarket shelves stacked with 'low fat' foods that are loaded with sugar. Fat makes the food more palatable; when you take it out, the food tastes like cardboard, so the food industry chose an additive that was cheap to mass produce and tasted good. One typical regular serving of fruit yogurt can contain up to six teaspoons of sugar!

Most recently, Canadian researchers carried out a huge analysis of all the data in order to find out whether there truly is an association between the consumption of saturated fat and heart disease. It looked at all relevant studies, which included those undertaken on over 300,000 healthy people followed for up to twenty-five years, and found no association between the consumption of saturated fat and any cause of death, heart attacks, heart-disease deaths, strokes or the development of type-2 diabetes.[3]

And this study was carried out not long after a very extensive analysis of 32 observational studies and 27 randomized controlled trials (RCT) involving over 630,000 participants undertaken by the Cambridge University Medical Research Council and funded by the British Heart Foundation which also found no association between saturated fat and heart disease. In addition, this research revealed that the consumption of a type of saturated fat found in dairy foods – margaric acid – was associated with *decreasing* the risk of heart disease.[4]

There has also been research done on people who have suffered a heart attack to see whether reducing saturated fat in their diet had any benefit. This concluded that doing so caused no reduction in heart attacks, strokes or death.[5]

The final nail in the coffin of attacks on saturated fat should have been a paper published in *Open Heart (British Medical Journal [BMJ])* by Harcombe et al.[6] This was the first of a series of papers from a fascinating PhD dissertation examining the evidence base for our total and saturated fat guidelines. It looked at randomized controlled evidence available to the dietary guideline committees at the time they introduced the 30 per cent total and 10 per cent saturated fat restrictions. Harcombe et al used systematic review and meta-analysis to show that the six RCTs available at the time did *not* support those guidelines. The evidence simply wasn't there. A further interesting finding from this paper was that the dietary fat interventions reduced cholesterol more than in the control groups and yet there was no difference in coronary heart disease mortality or mortality from any cause. Lower cholesterol made no difference whatsoever to number of deaths!

In October 2013, I wrote what turned out to be a widely publicized editorial in the *BMJ* entitled 'Saturated Fat is Not the Major Issue', which, in addition to throwing a cat among the pigeons at the time, led to the much-needed reignition of scientific debate around this issue.[7]

In addition, I suggested that we should be concentrating public-health efforts on sugar as the number-one villain in the western diet.

Although I didn't reference this in my editorial, one fascinating study, which was not well publicized, measured the progression of coronary-artery blockages in a group of postmenopausal women with diagnosed heart disease. This was done with a test called a coronary angiogram, which directly visualizes the heart arteries. I've performed well over a thousand of these myself. The researchers found that consumption of saturated fat was associated with a lower progression of blocked arteries over a number of years, in comparison to carbohydrate or polyunsaturated fats.[8]

How can all this be explained on a biological level? Doesn't saturated fat in the diet raise 'bad' cholesterol? Well, yes and no.

Of course, there will be variations from person to person in how their body responds to increases in saturated fat in their diet, but what tends to be consistent is that even if so-called bad cholesterol (LDL, or low-density lipoproteins) is raised, good cholesterol (HDL, or high-density lipoproteins) is also increased by saturated fat, which makes its overall effect on cardiovascular risk (the risk of suffering a heart attack or stroke in the next ten years) neutral. This is because it is the total cholesterol to HDL-C ratio that doctors use to calculate cardiovascular risk, not levels of LDL-C. Furthermore, if we look at LDL cholesterol in isolation, it is made up of two types of subparticles: type A, which are big and buoyant (think of a large balloon); and type B, which are small, dense particles thought to be much more likely to damage the heart arteries because of their greater ability to penetrate the inner lining of the coronary arteries. Saturated fats that increase LDL cholesterol in the blood have a preponderance to increase the large, buoyant particles, whereas the small, dense, more damaging particles increase in response to sugar and other refined carbohydrates in the diet.

As I reveal in *The Big Fat Fix*, when I personally added a daily tablespoon of coconut oil into my low-sugar, low-refined-carbohydrate diet and rechecked my cholesterol a few months later, my HDL had shot up much more than my LDL, which made my ratio and, therefore, my risk of suffering a heart attack in the next ten years slightly lower.

So, I think what we can say is that, when it comes to heart disease, at worst, saturated fat in the diet has a neutral effect (in other words, it's not harmful to the heart), and, at best, it may be protective if it comes from dairy products.

What about the people of Pioppi?

In the research that Donal and I carried out in the making of *The Big Fat Fix*, we did find that those in Pioppi didn't have a diet rich in dairy products other than cheese, but this wasn't out of choice; other dairy products simply weren't widely available during Ancel Keys's time. Nor did they eat a lot meat; it was expensive. Although they were unaware of it at the time, a diet with hardly any sugar and one that was rich in locally sourced vegetables and fish, with olive oil eaten with practically every meal, gave them significant health benefits. We'll come on to the bread and pasta a little later!

Is this an excuse to gorge on foods high in fat and saturated fat? Absolutely not. Once you have cut out the sugar and refined carbohydrates and your general daily food intake includes foods in which it's most likely that the benefits of the Mediterranean lie, then cooking in butter or coconut oil, which add such great flavour to food, and eating moderate amounts of cheese and other full-fat dairy foods which provide good nutritional value can be very much a part of a healthy diet.

In summary:

- The 90 per cent of increase in calories in the American diet between 1961 and 2011 has come from refined carbohydrates and industrial seed oils

- Fat in unprocessed food is a crucial provider of essential fats vital to health

- Dietary fat is satiating (i.e. it keeps you fuller for longer); refined carbohydrates and sugar aren't

- Dietary fat has the least impact on raising glucose and insulin

- Saturated fat does not clog the heart arteries

6.

Cholesterol: Friend or Foe?

'Cholesterol is an enormously complex
molecule, and to think that you can radically pull
this out of the body and not have consequences
is ridiculous. It's such bad science.'

– Dr John Abramson, Harvard School
of Public Health

For decades, it's been assumed that cholesterol is a toxic substance in the body and that getting your cholesterol as low as you can is good for your health, but, as I will explain, not only is this misleading, but also, this misunderstanding has had a considerable harmful effect on our overall health. And things are not helped by the fact that the media, and many scientists and doctors (under the financial influence of the food and pharmaceutical industry), still disseminate selected, biased and outdated information. But before we examine the totality of the science surrounding cholesterol, let's first gain a basic understanding of what it is.

Cholesterol is a fatty, wax-like substance that is present

in all cells of the body and has many important functions, including the production of the sex hormones oestrogen, testosterone and progesterone. Cholesterol helps produce bile acids, which help in the digestion and absorption of fat-soluble vitamins from the intestine into the bloodstream.

Cholesterol is also involved in the body's synthesis of vitamin D, which is essential for the maintenance of bone integrity. In addition, it has a crucial role in creating and sustaining the integrity of cell membranes. In other words, without cholesterol, we wouldn't be able to survive.

Eighty per cent of levels of blood cholesterol that is synthesized by the body is genetically predetermined, with the remaining 20 per cent influenced by diet. Because cholesterol cannot dissolve in water, it travels in a shell of proteins which is manufactured in the liver in order to fulfil its various functions in the body. These lipoproteins are low-density lipoproteins (LDL) or high-density lipoproteins (HDL); traditionally known as 'bad' and 'good' cholesterol, respectively. Another component of total cholesterol which is routinely measured in the blood are triglycerides. Triglycerides are the main constituents of body fat, and its metabolism also involves it being broken down to form glucose as a source of energy. Its metabolism and blood levels are also controlled by the liver.

So how did cholesterol and, more specifically, LDL cholesterol get such a bad name? One reason is Ancel Keys's Seven Countries Study linking high cholesterol and heart disease, but a landmark study launched in 1948 in the town of Framingham, Massachusetts, also contributed. More than 5,000 healthy men and women aged between thirty and sixty-two were initially studied, and the study is now looking at the third generation of the population.

There have been over a thousand medical publications linked to the study in Framingham and, from its results following up the participants, 'risk factors' for heart disease were determined and used to calculate the likelihood of an individual suffering a heart attack in the next ten years. The more risk factors, the greater the risk. Before the Framingham study was initiated, there were already hypotheses that heart disease could be explained by lifestyle factors, by the environment and by genetic predisposition. It was this study that identified smoking, high blood pressure and high cholesterol as major risk factors for heart disease.

It also threw up some interesting statistics that are not widely known or appreciated. For every 1mg/per decilitre drop in blood cholesterol levels, there was a 14 per cent increase in cardiovascular death and an 11 per cent increase in mortality in the following eighteen years in those aged over fifty.[1] Not only should this should have been a red flag to those pushing the cholesterol hypothesis, there were also some criticisms about how strongly one could attribute the characteristics of the Framingham population to other nationalities.

Another spanner in the works, which, however, did draw attention, came in 2001, when a heart study undertaken in Honolulu, Hawaii, and published in the *Lancet* looked at a group of elderly Japanese American men and also found an inverse association with total cholesterol and death, this time in those aged over seventy. The researchers concluded: 'We have been unable to explain our results. These data cast doubt on the scientific justification of lowering cholesterol to very low concentrations (less than 4.65mmol/L) in elderly people.'[2]

One of the reasons for this may be that HDL cholesterol is known to protect against heart attack and, as mentioned above, when doctors calculate cardiovascular risk (using the QRISK online calculator as well as other risk factors, such as type-2 diabetes, blood pressure and family history, it is the ratio of total cholesterol divided by HDL ratio that is used.

However, some questions about bad cholesterol, or LDL-C, remained unanswered.

In 2016, I and sixteen international researchers from five different countries (the UK, Sweden, Italy, Japan and the US) set out to look specifically at all the data on people over the age of sixty and find out what the correlation was between LDL-C and cardiovascular disease.

One of the reasons we focused on those over the age of sixty is that most people who suffer a heart attack are this age so, if LDL-C was strongly implicated in the development of heart disease, one would expect to find at least some association here.

What we found was quite extraordinary. Pooling together a number of studies looking at populations across the world, which included almost 70,000 people, we found that not only was there no association between LDL-C and cardiovascular disease but that there was an inverse association between LDL-C and all-cause mortality. In other words, if you are aged over sixty, the higher your LDL cholesterol, the less likely you were to die.[3]

How can this be explained biologically? What is little appreciated is that LDL also has an important role in the immune system and therefore may protect elderly people from acute infections such as pneumonia and stomach illnesses, which are a major cause of death in this age group.

Coming back to Framingham, another important finding was that there was very little difference in cholesterol levels between those who did and those who didn't develop heart disease, unless total cholesterol was very low (less than 150mg/decilitre USA units of measurement or 3.88mmol/litre UK units of measurement) or extremely high (more than 380mg/decilitre or 9.84 mmol/litre).[4]

And those historic findings are also consistent with the largest study carried out to date in the US, which examined over 130,000 patients being admitted to hospital with a heart attack and found that 75 per cent had normal total cholesterol and LDL levels. In this group, 66 per cent of patients fulfilled the criteria for metabolic syndrome; this was the most important risk factor.[5]

To meet the criteria, an individual patient must have any three of the following five conditions: impaired glucose tolerance or type-2 diabetes, raised blood pressure (greater than 140/90mmHg), high triglycerides (greater than 150mg/decilitre or greater than 1.7mmol/litre), low HDL cholesterol (less than 35mg/decilitre or 1.03 mmol/litre in men and less than 39mg/decilitre or 1.29 mmol/litre in women) and increased waist circumference (more than 90cm and 84cm for men and women, respectively). It was also later determined that, despite the best medical treatment, metabolic syndrome was an adverse prognostic indicator. In other words, if you had metabolic syndrome and suffered a heart attack, you were 50 per cent more likely either to be readmitted to hospital or to die within the following year.

The triglyceride to HDL ratio (which is rapidly responsive to dietary changes that involve cutting out refined carbohydrates and including healthy high-fat foods in the diet) is a much better predictor of heart-attack risk. An examination of the extent and severity of heart disease in a study of people undergoing coronary angiography and considered to be at high risk found that the triglyceride to HDL ratio was the best predictor of how much disease was present. Yet again, in this study, which directly examined the heart arteries, there was no significant relationship between the extent of heart disease and total cholesterol or LDL-C.[6]

But what about dietary trials and drugs trials designed to lower cholesterol? Don't they reduce heart attacks and death rates?

None of the dietary trials (the best-quality scientific evidence to demonstrate cause and effect) that lowered total and LDL cholesterol through dietary changes (i.e. a reduction in saturated fat) have shown a reduction in the incidence of heart attack, stroke or death. And this was the case even before the introduction of the change in dietary guidelines advising us to cut down on saturated fat in 1977 and 1983 in the US and UK, respectively.

In addition, a research paper published in the *British*

Medical Journal in 2016 revealed that efforts to reduce total and LDL cholesterol may actually have a detrimental effect. Re-analysis of unpublished data from the famous Sydney diet heart study and the Minnesota coronary experiment showed that patients with heart disease who replaced saturated fat with vegetable oils high in omega-6 fats showed increased heart-attack and death rates, despite significant reductions in total and LDL cholesterol.[7]

And, other than statin drugs, no other cholesterol-lowering drug has been demonstrated to have any impact on reducing death rates from heart disease, and, even with statins, many patients when told the absolute benefit in terms of living longer find them particularly underwhelming. For example, if you are diagnosed with heart disease or have suffered a heart attack, there's a one in eighty-three chance that taking a statin every day for five years will delay your death and a one in thirty-nine chance that it will prevent or delay another heart attack.[8] But if you haven't suffered a heart attack or haven't been diagnosed with heart disease, it will not prolong your life by one day.[9]

And the above probably represents the very best case scenario because many individuals – possibly, up to a third – are removed from the clinical trials before they even begin, for various reasons, including not being able to tolerate taking the drug due to its side effects that interfere with the quality of life.[10]

Given all the data we now have available, it is far more plausible that the benefit from statin drugs in reducing heart-attack rates derive from their effects on reducing inflammation.

Even Ancel Keys, towards the end of his life, appeared to acknowledge that the low-cholesterol bandwagon had gone off the tracks, being quoted in the *New York Times* in 1987 as saying, 'I've come to believe that cholesterol is not as important [as a risk factor for heart attacks] as we used to think it was.'[11]

What can we conclude from all this? Firstly, LDL cholesterol is not the bogeyman it's been portrayed to be. It's the LDL particle size that has a stronger association with heart disease and is more atherogenic (prone to damaging the inner lining of the coronary artery). Secondly, putting total cholesterol and LDL cholesterol to the top of the list of targets to prevent and treat heart disease is sorely misguided. Professor Rita Redberg sums it up perfectly. In addition to being a world-respected professor of cardiology at the University of California, San Francisco, she is also editor in chief of medical journal *JAMA Internal Medicine*. She says, 'Cholesterol is just a lab number. Who cares about lowering cholesterol unless it actually translates into a benefit for patients?'

So, instead of fearing cholesterol, we need to make it our friend by improving its profile to reduce the risk of cardiovascular disease. Even better, once one focuses on the elephant in the room – the real root cause of heart disease – then the cholesterol will take care of itself.

In summary:

- Cholesterol is one of the most vital molecules in the body; without it, we would die

- If you're over sixty years old, high **LDL** cholesterol is not associated with cardiovascular disease and is inversely associated with mortality from any cause

- 75 per cent of people admitted with a heart attack have normal total and **LDL** cholesterol, but 66 per cent have metabolic syndrome

- The triglyceride to **HDL** ratio is a much better predictor of heart-attack risk than total cholesterol or **LDL** cholesterol

- If you haven't had a heart attack, and you don't suffer with heart disease, taking a cholesterol-lowering statin pill will not prolong your life by one day

7.

The Root Cause of Heart Disease: Insulin Resistance and Inflammation

'I think the condition we're dealing with
that encompasses all these diseases – heart
disease, high blood pressure, dementia and
even cancer – is insulin resistance.'

– Professor Timothy Noakes

Insulin is a hormone produced by the pancreas; the primary role of which helps cells in the body to take up blood glucose to be used as energy. As glucose goes up, insulin goes up. It also has many other functions, which involve converting excess glucose that is not immediately used for energy into glycogen for storage, protein synthesis and fat metabolism. By converting excess glucose into triglycerides to be stored as fat, insulin also prevents the breakdown of stored fat to be used as energy. Many therefore refer to insulin as the 'fat-storing' hormone.

Insulin resistance occurs when the body's liver, muscle and fat cells become resistant to the effects of insulin, causing the pancreas to secrete more and more insulin to compensate. Eventually, the blood glucose level rises above the normal range, which then leads to a diagnosis of type-2 diabetes. However, insulin resistance (a marker of which is chronically raised insulin levels, or hyper-insulinaemia) itself can be present for many years, even decades, before an individual is diagnosed with type-2 diabetes. (I'll discuss this in more detail in Chapter 8.)

Insulin resistance has also been shown to be a power-ful independent predictor of strokes, high blood pressure, cancer and heart disease.[1] In 2009, the journal *Diabetes Care* published a paper containing the results of a math-ematical analysis of the hierarchy of risk factors for heart attacks. It estimated that, if these risk factors were addressed in men aged between twenty and thirty, then a significant proportion of heart attacks would be pre-vented in the future. At the top of this list was insulin resistance. According to the calculations, and taking into consideration some overlap, correcting insulin resistance alone would prevent 42 per cent of all heart attacks; cor-recting high blood pressure, 36 per cent of all heart attacks; correcting low HDL cholesterol, 31 per cent; cor-recting high body mass index, 21 per cent; correcting high LDL cholesterol, 16 per cent; and correcting high trigly-cerides, 10 per cent.[2]

They concluded, 'Insulin resistance is likely the single most important cause of CAD (coronary artery disease). A better understanding of its pathogenesis and how it could be prevented or cured could have a profound effect on CAD.' Notice that LDL cholesterol comes pretty low on the list. And, given what we know about atherogenic dyslipidaemia (characterized by high triglycerides, low HDL cholesterol and raised small, dense LDL cholesterol particles), it is very likely this benefit was related to correcting for raised LDL type-B subparticles, which, you will remember from Chapter 6, are increased by the consumption of refined carbohydrates and sugar.

Dr Joseph Kraft also identified insulin resistance (hyperinsulinaemia) as the number-one driver of heart disease. In an illustrious career as both a physician and a pathologist which spanned decades, Kraft found that the overwhelming majority of those with heart disease – well over 80 per cent – had hyperinsulinaemia. He created a test that picks up hyperinsulinaemia well before blood-glucose ranges measured in the traditional way become abnormal and are diagnosed as in the prediabetic or diabetes ranges. He verified the work of the famed pathologist Kimmelstiel, who showed that diabetic kidney damage occurred long before glucose abnormalities become apparent in patients. Kraft extended Kimmelstiel's findings. He discovered that the damage to blood vessels of the heart occurs much earlier than the usual measure of blood glucose would categorize it as falling outside the normal range. He termed this 'diabetes in situ'. As he puts it, 'Those with cardiovascular disease not identified with diabetes are simply undiagnosed.' There is a considerable overlap with metabolic syndrome and insulin resistance, of which a high triglyceride to HDL ratio (more than 2.75 in men and more than 1.65 in women) is highly predictive of metabolic syndrome. This ratio is also highly correlated with the risk of suffering a heart attack, irrespective of BMI.[3]

Insulin resistance is also closely associated with markers of the metabolic syndrome, which, as I explained in Chapter 6, is present in the majority of those admitted with a heart attack. But, more importantly, this also holds for a significant proportion of those of 'normal' weight. In fact, it is estimated that up to 40 per cent of those with a normal BMI have markers of the metabolic syndrome. And this also fits in with my own observations, having treated thousands of patients with heart disease in the course of my career. In other words, there is no such thing as a 'healthy weight'; we should instead focus on what makes a healthy person.

So, despite the wealth of scientific data at our disposal, why is so little known about insulin resistance, and why isn't it more widely discussed? Well, one of the reasons is that we are using outdated concepts and flawed science ('low fat is good', 'eat less, move more', 'maintain a healthy weight', and so on), and this is compounded by the conventional medical model of treating risk factors or symptoms with drugs (which have marginal benefits at best, and have side effects) while simultaneously failing to address the root causes of ill health.

We have focused, wrongly, on the quantity of cholesterol measured in the bloodstream, and consequently on lowering it with diet and drugs, as if was an end in itself. What we have neglected to do is to look at the *quality* of cholesterol. These incorrect beliefs, along with commercially driven bad science and finance-based medicine, have, unfortunately, led many people to think that they can gorge on junk food without suffering any adverse effects, as long as they're taking statins. This illusion of protection will ultimately result in far more harm to individuals' health. And, last but not least, up until now, no market or business model has been created to spread the message about a risk factor that can be prevented, or at least rapidly attenuated, by making simple lifestyle changes.

Insulin has such an important role in the metabolism of fat and glucose that, when its function is dysregulated by chronically high insulin, it sets up a vicious cycle of excess fat accumulation in the liver and, in addition, stops fat being oxidized (burned for energy) by reducing the levels of an important protein called adiponectin. Low adiponectin is inversely correlated with visceral fat, that is, fat that accumulates around organs in the abdominal cavity, specifically, the pancreas, intestines and liver. An insulin-resistant liver will churn more glucose and triglycerides into the bloodstream, and this usually goes hand in hand with low HDL cholesterol. It is visceral fat that is responsible for increased waist circumference, which is a much better marker for metabolic health, total body fat and risk of future health problems than body mass index. Some surveys in England have revealed that an increase in BMI tends to flatten out in older age, but waist circumference is still growing by eight to ten centimetres every ten years, well into people reaching their seventies. The reason for this is that as muscle mass declines in older age, especially in those who are not active, there's an increase in body fatness, which is not picked up by BMI. Bigger waists and loss of muscle (known as sarcopenic obesity) leads to a higher incidence of type-2 diabetes, physical disability and falls and fractured hips in older people.

Moving on from the evils of insulin resistance, we now turn to its twin brother, chronic inflammation. There is a lot of overlap between the two, as one drives the other. The more insulin resistance in an individual's body, the more systemic inflammation, and vice versa.

When an individual has an infection or suffers an injury, the body's immune and inflammatory response protects them; this is an acute inflammatory reaction and is life-saving. Chronic inflammation, however, is not. Imagine the body being under constant attack from environmental stimuli such as smoking, poor diet and stress. This brings us on to the real underlying cause of heart disease.

Coronary artery disease often manifests when the blood flow in one or more of the vessels that supply the heart muscle with blood becomes restricted. This restriction happens as the result of a build-up of plaque or narrowings in the vessel wall over time (a process known as atherosclerosis).

For a patient, this may present as a symptom of chest discomfort that comes on with exercise (usually when the blood vessel is narrowed by more than 70 per cent). Often, however, it is first diagnosed when the individual suffers a heart attack. A heart attack occurs when part of the heart muscle is deprived of oxygen for a long enough period for cell death to occur.

Traditionally, it was thought that narrowings progress over time until the vessel becomes completely (100 per cent) blocked and that was the cause of heart attack. But this rarely happens. In fact, more than 50 per cent of those who suffer a first heart attack have no preceding symptoms. We now understand that most heart attacks happen at sites where the narrowing is less than 70 per cent. How can this be explained? An atherosclerosis begins with damage to the inner lining of the coronary arteries: a combination of inflammatory and immune cells from the blood, together with cholesterol, migrate into the vessel wall. Over time (generally over decades, as the initial minor fatty streaks have been discovered at autopsy in young men killed in war), this can enlarge and encroach on the lumen (the inside of the vessel), causing angina, or suddenly occlude (block the blood flow), which can be visualized in terms of a 'pimple' bursting.[4]

When this pimple bursts (in medical terms, we call this plaque rupture), clotting factors are released to the site which can completely block the blood flow to the heart muscle and cause a heart attack. The sooner the blood supply is restored through treatment with a drug such as aspirin which acts as a blood thinner, and a keyhole surgical procedure to mechanically dislodge the clot (primary angioplasty) is undertaken, the less damage to heart muscle and the lower the risk of death.

There's something very interesting about this procedure. Although unblocking the artery by means of mechanical manipulation by using a small balloon and deploying a metal coil known as a stent (a small metal scaffold) can be life-saving while someone is suffering a heart attack, it doesn't prevent one. In other words, if someone is diagnosed with angina and found to have a 70 per cent or greater narrowing, stretching the artery by inflating a small balloon at the site and implanting a stent that stays there permanently to improve blood flow has been consistently proven *not* to prevent heart attacks or prolong life.[5]

That may sound counterintuitive, but it isn't when one understands that non-severe plaques are more vulnerable to rupture, that the stent is not actually removing the blockage and it can occlude and cause a heart attack that may otherwise never have happened. However, most importantly, stents do not address the underlying cause: inflammation.

Another fascinating aspect is the heart's ability to adapt to a gradual build-up of blockages by forming extra, small, protective blood vessels that compensate and bypass the blockage. These are known as collaterals. I have seen, on numerous occasions, patients who have undergone coronary angiograms after complaining of angina symptoms where one of the three major coronary arteries is completely blocked but there's no evidence of any previous damage to heart muscle. Usually, one of the two other arteries has grown new small vessels to make up for the area of heart muscle previously supplied with blood from the now blocked major artery.

To summarize, coronary artery disease is actually a chronic inflammatory disease in which the immune system interacts with metabolic risk factors to commence and enhance the build-up of narrowings in the heart arteries which become prone to suddenly forming clots which lead to a heart attack. Its prevention and treatment, therefore, must involve interventions that will help reduce this inflammation.

And this risk can rapidly be reduced by stopping smoking, making changes to one's diet, engaging in mindful movement and reducing stress. In other words, by following the Pioppi Diet!

Let's start with smoking.

Although cardiovascular disease (heart attacks and strokes) still remains the number-one cause of premature death in European men, and the biggest causes of death worldwide (approximately 20 million deaths a year), 50 per cent of the decline in death rates from a heart attack in the western world in the past three decades can be attributed purely to a reduction in tobacco consumption across the population. And the single most rapid impact appeared to occur after public smoking bans were instituted. Here are two well-documented examples.

In 2002, Helena, the capital city of Montana, in the US, within six months of the introduction of a ban on smoking in public places there was a 40 per cent decline in hospital admissions of patients suffering a heart attack.[6] When the law was rescinded, admission rates went back to their previous levels. Similarly, a few years later, when a public smoking ban was introduced in Scotland, there was a 17 per cent reduction of such hospital admissions within a year and a 6 per cent fall in the number of those dying outside hospital from cardiac arrest. How can such a dramatic effect be explained? Remember my explanation of plaque rupture? As it turns out, just thirty minutes of passive smoking increases platelet activity (platelets are the blood cells involved in clotting).[7] In other words, removing one's exposure to smoke in the environment reduces the stickiness of the blood, making it less likely to clot and so contribute to the occlusion of the blood vessel.

Another fascinating statistic when one compares the significantly higher death rates from coronary disease in the US, compared to Mediterranean countries, fifty years ago – around the time Ancel Keys was conducting his Seven Countries Study – is that the average American was consuming twice the number of cigarettes consumed by the average citizen in southern Europe.

In Chapter 6, I explained that randomized trials designed to reduce cholesterol through diet had no effect on improving important health outcomes, and in some cases had the opposite effect. So, have there been any good-quality studies that have been proven to reduce the incidence of heart attacks, strokes and premature death from related causes? And does the evidence suggest that the adoption of specific dietary patterns and foods has such a rapid effect in reducing heart attacks as giving up smoking? The answer is a big YES. There have been several randomized controlled trials, looking at both primary and secondary prevention.

Primary prevention means an intervention undertaken in order to prevent a disease from occurring (so in those who have not yet had a heart attack). Secondary prevention is the management of a disease once it has been diagnosed in order to prevent further adverse consequences (so to prevent those who survive a heart attack from having another one).

Let's first discuss a landmark primary prevention trial.

The PREDIMED study was a trial funded by the Spanish government that compared two Mediterranean diets in approximately 7,500 middle-aged participants considered to be at high risk of cardiovascular disease. The trial had a good split of men (43 per cent) and women (57 per cent). The trial tested a higher-fat Mediterranean diet against a lower-fat traditional Mediterranean diet. The latter group was specifically told to reduce consumption of all types of fat, with an emphasis on eating more low-fat dairy products, lean meat, potatoes, pasta, rice, fruit and vegetables.

The hypothesis under examination was whether an intake of at least four tablespoons of extra virgin olive oil daily, or a handful of tree nuts (15g walnuts, 7.5g almonds and 7.5g hazelnuts), compared to the lower-fat diet, would provide any benefit in reducing rates of heart attack, stroke or death.

After a follow-up of almost five years, the trial was terminated because it became clear that there was a significant benefit in the higher-fat Mediterranean diet groups, which showed 30 per cent fewer cardiovascular events (heart attacks, strokes or death). Further statistical analysis revealed that this was due primarily to a reduction in the incidence of strokes.[8]

The trial also had some other important features. The first was that it was 'energy unrestricted'; in other words, there was no calorie counting. I'll discuss the rationale behind this in Chapter 9. The second was that there was no significant difference in cholesterol between the two groups – but that should no longer surprise you. The third was the rapidity of the benefits of the diet in reducing stroke rates started to occur within a period of weeks. These foods were, in effect, medicine.

And, last but not least, the diet of those following the low-fat diet was still quite healthy in comparison to the average western diet, as they were also advised to eat plenty of vegetables and to cut down on sweets. In other words, it is highly probable that if the Mediterranean Diet, supplemented with extra virgin olive oil or nuts, was compared to the typical western diet of processed and fast food, the results would have been even more spectacular.

Other previous studies have revealed that eating fast food more than twice a week doubles insulin resistance, and that the consumption of trans fats (traditionally found in fried and packaged foods, such as ready-made meals, cakes and biscuits) increases C-reactive protein and other markers of inflammation in the blood within weeks. Luckily, the addition of industrial trans fats in packaged foods has dramatically declined in western countries in the past fifteen to twenty years, and this has also significantly contributed to a reduction in death rates from cardiovascular disease in the population. It's estimated that the banning of trans fats from the food supply in 2004 has prevented 7,000 cardiovascular deaths in Denmark over ten years.[9]

Since the PREDIMED trial was terminated in 2013,

those who adopted the higher-fat Mediterranean diet have been followed up, and the further analysis of improvements in their health have been quite extraordinary. Of the over 4,000 women recruited in the trial, those who were consuming at least four tablespoons of extra virgin olive oil on top of the traditional diet had a 68 per cent lower risk of breast cancer, relative to those advised to follow the low-fat diet over a period of five years. Researchers undertaking a separate analysis of the PREDIMED participants found in addition that there was less cognitive decline in those consuming a handful of nuts every day. However, this is not new to the Mediterranean diet in general. Ahead of the G8 summit on dementia in December 2013, myself and a number of eminent UK and international doctors wrote a letter to then prime minister David Cameron and the Secretary of State for Health urging them to make the Mediterranean diet central to policy in tackling dementia, a condition which now costs western economies $420 billion per annum.

In the letter, we stated that this was all the more important because drugs to slow the progression of dementia are of dubious value, are extremely costly and have side effects. One significant twenty-year study looked at middle-aged people (those between the ages of forty-three and sixty-four) who adopted a Mediterranean dietary pattern, and found that those with the highest adherence to this pattern had significantly less decline in memory function into old age. These findings were consistent even accounting for differing levels of physical activity and whether or not they smoked. A separate analysis of other studies revealed that those who adopt a Mediterranean diet at the early stages of Alzheimer's experienced a slowing of the deterioration in their memory. So, not only does a Mediterranean diet prevent the onset of dementia, it also helps reduce the deterioration in the condition in those suffering from it.

In addition to protecting the brain from the damage associated with dementia, omega-3 fatty acids and anti-inflammatory properties in nuts, oily fish, olive oil and a variety of vegetables also improve cerebral blood flow (as demonstrated by brain MRI scans).

The PREDIMED study indicated that the greatest benefit of the Mediterranean diet was in preventing strokes; however, a landmark study published in 2017 revealed that the beneficial effects on the brain also appear to extend to the prevention of depression.[10]

This study, carried out by researchers in Australia, revealed that a Mediterranean diet which was low in sugar and refined cereals and pasta significantly improved mood in patients with severe depression within just twelve weeks. The lead researcher, Professor Felice Jacka, Director of Deakin University's Food and Mood Centre, told ABC News Australia, 'We already know that diet has a very potent impact on the biological aspects of our body that affect depression risks. The immune system, brain plasticity and gut microbiota seem to be central not just to our physical health but also our mental health.'

There's been a lot of interest in the gut microbiome recently, so we'll touch on it very briefly here. The term 'microbiome' (or 'microbiota') refers to the trillions of microbes and bacteria that reside in our gut which can now be easily tested using genetic methods. We are now beginning to understand that these microbes are essential for brain development, as well as being heavily involved in the regulation of the immune system and metabolism. The microbiota are also involved in the production of the hormone serotonin, which, when depleted, can lead to depression. Environmental and processed food chemicals that wipe out the good bacteria from our gut and reduce diversity have been linked to the development of many disorders including obesity, depression, allergies, autoimmune diseases and the metabolic syndrome. Artificial sweeteners, antibiotics and lack of fibre appear to have a negative effect on the gut microbiome.

Professor Tim Spector, a genetic epidemiologist at King's College London (and author of *The Diet Myth*), has done extensive research in this area, and it turns out that several foods, many of which are considered to be part of the traditional Mediterranean diet, appear to be beneficial to the gut and increase diversity. These include foods that are rich in fibre or polyphenols, such as a variety of non-starchy vegetables, nuts, seeds, olive oil, onions, garlic, dark chocolate, coffee, red wine, certain cheeses and fermented foods such as live yogurt, kefir and kimchi. And indeed it is precisely these types of food, predominantly in the form of locally sourced vegetables, that we discovered were key staples in the diet of the residents of Pioppi.

Let's move on to secondary prevention of cardiovascular disease. Can changing your diet after you have suffered a heart attack prevent further heart attacks or prolong life?

Published in the *Lancet* in 1994 (as a preliminary report) and 1999 (in its final version) the Lyon Diet Heart Study was a randomized controlled trial of more than 600 survivors of a first heart attack. One group was given the standard American Heart Association (AHA) recommended 'low fat' diet, and the comparison group consumed a Mediterranean diet rich in olive oil and with a liberal use of rapeseed margarine. Rapeseed is similar in composition to olive oil but has significantly more omega-3 fatty acids. The results seen in the Mediterranean diet group were quite extraordinary. There was a 70 per cent risk reduction in cardiovascular complications by the end of four years, relative to the American Heart Association diet.

To put this in perspective, for every thirty people adopting the Mediterranean diet rather than the AHA recommended diet, one life was saved. The impact on reducing death rates was almost three times as powerful as taking a statin drug (one in eighty-three), and there were no side effects. The reduction in further heart attacks was even more significant, at one in eighteen, but there was another surprising finding: there was a significantly lower rate in the onset of cancer after four years (one in thirty people).

Again, there was no difference in cholesterol levels between the two groups, which suggests that something else in the diet was having a beneficial effect. By now, it should be clear that it's the anti-inflammatory components (polyphenols) of the foods that are important, but another major factor also appeared to play a significant role: the omega-6 to omega-3 fatty acid ratio.

Dr Artemis Simopoulos, founder of the Center of Genetics, Nutrition and Health, in Washington DC, has conducted extensive research on the impact of the omega-6 to omega-3 ratio on health. An imbalance of these essential fatty acids has been associated with heart disease, colorectal cancer, breast cancer and rheumatoid arthritis. Our hunter-gatherer ancestors in the Paleolithic period had a ratio of almost 1:1; in modern western diets, the ratio is closer to 25:1. Simopoulos points out that the Paleolithic ratio was also the average ratio of the population of the Greek island of Crete during the time Ancel Keys conducted his Seven Countries Study. Crete at that time had the lowest mortality rate from coronary heart disease and any cause of death than any other Mediterranean region, despite similar levels of cholesterol.[11]

Simopoulos points out that the typical Cretan diet consisted predominantly of a high intake of fruits, vegetables, legumes, nuts, olive oil and olives, cheese and fish, of sourdough bread rather than pasta, and less meat.

Eggs and meat came from grazing poultry and animals; modern western farmed, grain-fed animal produce is deficient in omega-3. In Crete, there was a perfect balance of omega-3 to omega-6 fatty acids throughout the food chain. There was also a high intake of selenium, a trace mineral with antioxidant properties. Selenium is found in abundance in foods such as octopus, yellowfin tuna, grass-fed beef and eggs. The Lyon Diet Heart Study (ratio 1:4) was in effect a modified version of the Cretan diet. Its beneficial components were used later to study a group of Indian patients with heart disease.

India has a very high rate of premature (under the age of sixty-five) death from cardiovascular disease, and this has increased in the past two decades. This is attributable to a combination of factors, including smoking and a rocketing prevalence of type-2 diabetes (India is second only to China in the world league). Unless this is brought under control, it's estimated that these premature deaths will cost the Indian economy $3 trillion by 2030. However, these known risk factors don't appear to be the only explanation. The typical ratio of omega-6 to omega-3 fats in rural India is pretty good, at 5–6:1, but in urban India it's closer to 40:1.

Many believe that it's not just individual components of the Mediterranean diet but in the synergy of the foods when eaten together that the added benefits lie. For example, olive oil increases the uptake of omega-3 fatty acids into the cell membrane, whereas the omega-6 from corn oil (used in the control American Heart Association diet of the Lyon Diet Heart Study) competes with the uptake.

Remember: omega-6 is also an essential fatty acid, as it plays a role in the immune response to infections. The problem in the western diet is getting too much of it from processed foods and also not getting enough omega-3.[12]

So which are the largest food sources of omega-6 fatty acids that send the balance in the wrong direction?

The answer is, essentially, anything that's been cooked in industrial seed oils, commonly known as vegetable oils, that is, corn oil, sunflower oil, safflower oil, soybean and cottonseed oil. This includes many baked goods, such as bread, cakes and pastries. But the problem isn't just with omega-6. Recent research carried out by chemical pathologist Professor Martin Grootveld from De Montford University in Leicester has revealed that, when these oils are heated to high temperatures, they form compounds called aldehydes which are linked to cancer, heart disease and dementia. A typical meal of fish and chips fried in such oils can contain aldehydes that are 100–200 times the limit recommended by the World Health Organization.[13] I personally avoid eating anything cooked in these oils, and when I occasionally venture into an Indian restaurant, if they're not able to cook my food in butter or ghee (which also tastes better), I don't eat there.

High blood pressure is traditionally considered the number-one risk factor for death globally, mainly because it is the number-one risk factor for strokes and is also a risk factor for heart attacks. Studies of populations reveal a significant increase in the risk of having a stroke after an individual's blood pressure goes above 140/90. It is estimated that one in three adult Americans suffer from high blood pressure. And it is estimated that 50 per cent of high blood pressure is caused by insulin resistance. Why not just take a pill to control it? Blood-pressure pills in the right group of patients have an important role in the prevention of strokes and heart attacks, but they appear to have the greatest benefit in those with the highest blood pressure, averaging above 160/100. An extensive analysis conducted by scientists of the Cochrane Collaboration pooling together randomized controlled trials involving 500,000 patients revealed that, in patients treated with drugs for mildly raised blood pressure (probably the majority on treatment in the UK), heart attacks, strokes and premature death were not prevented, despite the fact that their blood pressure had been brought down.[14]

It's difficult to explain why this may be the case but, as with many drugs, there may be unintended and other unknown effects on the body that cancel out any benefit from lowering blood pressure. It could also be related to the fact that almost one in ten individuals on treatment (9 per cent) suffer unacceptable side effects. However, perhaps most importantly, it may be because the underlying cause in half of these cases – insulin resistance – is not being addressed. I have seen a number of patients who, within weeks of changing their lifestyle, primarily by cutting out sugar and refined carbohydrates, have seen their mildly raised blood pressures drop into the normal range, even without increasing their level of physical activity.

If these patients did increase their level of physical activity just a little, they would probably have experienced further benefits. In a study of sedentary middle-aged adults, just thirty minutes of brisk walking three times a week helped reverse insulin resistance within months, even if they had not lost weight. Walking briskly for at least 150 minutes a week can increase average life expectancy by 3.2 years. And this is consistent with the lifestyle of the residents of Pioppi, where there isn't a gym. Their regular form of activity is walking outside.

And it's not just diet and regular activity that has an

effect on insulin resistance and chronic inflammation. Sleep and social cohesion are very powerful lifestyle factors with implications for our health, but they are often overlooked.

The power of quality sleep is profound. Everybody knows this. Whereas food choices can ignite fanatical (almost religious, in some cases) enthusiasm, you will rarely, if ever, engage in or even overhear a debate on sleep. The funny thing is, we all know this without recourse to any scientific research.

In fact, the research on sleep is very limited by comparison to that on drugs, exercise and other more lucrative pharmaceutical or health-related phenomena. The market for sleeping pills on the internet is enormous simply because, if you aren't getting enough quality sleep, the consequences are such that you will quickly take steps to try to remedy the situation.

We know that just one night of poor sleep makes you less insulin sensitive the following day. Evidence points to seven hours as a minimum recommendation to reap the powerful benefits of a good night's sleep. That lowered insulin sensitivity is not an isolated hormonal incident either. Testosterone has been shown to slide, cognitive performance diminishes and our hunger-signalling hormone – ghrelin – can start playing tricks on us.

In short, after one night of restricted or broken sleep, we may perform poorly all round and have a greater propensity to make poor 'pick me up' food choices throughout the day. It is no surprise that several consecutive days of restricted sleep has been proven to reduce performance significantly. That's around Thursday in the average working week. Sound familiar?

The afternoon siesta in Pioppi has been a daily fixture of life in that region for a very, very long time. These people intuitively know the importance of sleep, and we are convinced that this is a key component of the *diaita* which has been completely ignored – until now. A siesta every day, seven days a week, 365 days a year? If only! Siestas may not be at all practical for the rest of us, but we can certainly take steps to improve the quality of the sleep we do get.

In addition, blue light from modern tech equipment can be devastatingly disruptive to melatonin levels in the body. If we are constantly disrupting the body's sleep signal, how can we expect anything but a poor outcome? Our phones, computers and iPads are causing a mini-jetlag effect when we use them habitually after dark. You may know what time it is, but your body will be tricked by the artificial blue light they emit.

To counter this, quit the habit altogether and/or install the excellent free Flux app on your devices – https://just-getflux.com/ – or consider a pair of blue-light-filter glasses (there are many options available online).

Social isolation is another lifestyle challenge which is now affecting more and more of the young, as well as the elderly. Lack of social interaction doesn't just increase the risk of mental-health problems and depression, it also significantly increases the risk of premature death from heart disease and cancer. It's estimated that severe loneliness in England affects 700,000 men and 1.1 million women over the age of fifty, and that it is as potent a cause of early death as smoking fifteen cigarettes a day.

In addition to plausible associations with alcohol, suicide and increasing drug use which contributes to ill health, biological changes are brought on by chronic exposure to stress associated with social isolation and these have a negative impact on the immune, neuroendocrine and cardiovascular system, inducing greater production of markers of inflammation in the blood.

Social interaction is also crucial to feelings of well-being and happiness. In his book *Happier*, Lecturer on Positive Psychology at Harvard Dr Tal Ben-Shahar, writes, 'Having people about whom we care and who care about us to share our lives with – to share the thoughts and feelings in our lives – intensifies our experience of meaning, consoles us in our pain, deepens our sense of delight in the world. "Without friendship," writes Aristotle, "no happiness is possible."'

Major childhood trauma can lower life expectancy by as much as twenty years. In their *Nature* editorial 'Too Toxic to Ignore', Nobel laureate in physiology Elizabeth Blackburn and Professor of Psychology Elissa Epel describe the shortening of human telomeres (genes involved in ageing and normal cell division) in response to failure to alleviate stress. This in turn is strongly linked to cardiovascular disease, type-2 diabetes, dementia and certain cancers. Some of their original research also revealed that the longer a mother had spent being the main carer for a chronically ill child, the shorter were her telomeres. The most psychologically distressed mothers had the shortest telomere lengths – the equivalent of ten years of ageing. But the good news is that there's evidence that it's never too late to have an impact on telomeres. Just three months of stress-reduction interventions such as meditation, Pilates or yoga, combined with changing one's diet and doing the right type of regular activity, can reduce telomere attrition and may even slow down the ageing process.[15]

One fascinating randomized controlled trial conducted in India on forty-two men with established heart disease revealed not only reduced progression of coronary artery stenosis (narrowing) in a group which adopted yoga, but also a regression of stenosis in comparison to the control group following a regime of standard care with control of risk factors for heart disease. In other words, there was evidence of reversal of heart disease from yoga and these benefits were seen after only one year![16]

In Pioppi, we were able to observe an overwhelming feeling of community and sense the warmth among the people. The elderly still walk together in groups and sit together, chatting and laughing, taking their time to savour delicious food soaked in the best locally sourced extra virgin olive oil while sipping on a glass of red wine. Within just a few days in the company of these extraordinary people, combined with the serene environment of the tiny Italian village, I found the chronic stress levels I had been experiencing for months dissipating. As it turns out, the far from affluent residents of Pioppi have stumbled on the secrets to health, happiness and longevity, something that not even the most expensive and best of western medicine has come anywhere close to matching.

In summary:

- Insulin is the 'fat storing hormone'

- Insulin resistance has been shown to be an independent risk factor for stroke, high blood pressure and cancer and the number-one risk factor for heart attack

- Forty per cent of people with a normal BMI have the same metabolic abnormalities as those with the metabolic syndrome

- Waist circumference is a more reliable marker for metabolic health than BMI

- Coronary artery disease is a chronic inflammatory condition, the risk of which can be rapidly reduced by lifestyle changes such as stopping smoking, changing diet, mindful movement and stress reduction

8.

Type-2 Diabetes is Carbohydrate-Intolerance Disease

'Having cut the carbs, I've seen patients reverse
their type-2 diabetes within three months. There's
no medication that does that.'

– Dr Neville Wellington, General Practitioner,
Cape Town, South Africa

She walked into my consultation room smiling. She was an Asian lady in her early sixties and was accompanied by her daughter. She had come to ask for a cardiac consultation because she had changed her diet after seeing me discuss type-2 diabetes as a condition of carbohydrate intolerance in an interview on the TV news. What she had done of her own accord as a consequence of seeing that interview was quite remarkable. She had been diagnosed with type-2 diabetes over twenty-five years previously, and having followed medical advice and adopting a low-fat, high-carbohydrate diet, her blood sugars gradually crept up, not surprisingly. From her initial prescription of tablets, she'd been on daily insulin injections for the past two decades, taking a whopping eighty units a day.

Within just three months of cutting out refined sugar, bread and rice and replacing it with more cheese and butter and fibrous vegetables, she no longer needed insulin. Although her blood sugars were now well under control from cutting out all refined carbohydrates, she was concerned that increasing saturated fat in her diet might now increase her risk of heart disease. Not only was I able to reassure her that foods such as milk, eggs, cheese and yogurt were not going to clog her heart arteries, her cholesterol profile had in fact slightly improved when it was repeated three months after she had made the changes to her diet.

Although her total cholesterol remained unchanged and her LDL hadn't budged, her triglycerides had gone down and her HDL had increased. Because of high average blood sugars over the years, her kidney function had in the last few years started to deteriorate and she was now in the range of mild kidney failure.

Type-2 diabetes is a multi-organ, multi-system disease that affects every major organ in the body. It is formally diagnosed when there is a fasting blood glucose above 7mmol/litre, or an HbA1C of greater than 6.5mmol/litre. Once diagnosed, the condition is associated with a significant increase in the risk of having problems relating to the large blood vessels, which can lead to heart disease, a stroke and peripheral vascular disease.

In over fifteen years as a qualified doctor, I've

witnessed up close the devastation caused to individuals and their families by this condition. Average life expectancy of those diagnosed as having type-2 diabetes is reduced by between five and fifteen years. One of my earliest, most memorable experiences was during my first year as a junior doctor working in Edinburgh Royal Infirmary. A man in his late fifties with type-2 diabetes who also happened to be a heavy smoker (the worst combination) was admitted with gangrene in his foot, a result of blocked blood vessels in his leg. The only way to stop it travelling further up his body and infecting his bloodstream, and to save his life, was to amputate. I'll never forget the sound as I and my senior colleague stood for several minutes either side of the anaesthetized man, sawing through bone and flesh.

Type-2 diabetes also significantly increases the risk of microvascular complications (disease of the smaller blood vessels), which affect the kidneys (nephropathy), the nerves (neuropathy) and the eyes (retinopathy).

And it doesn't stop there: quality of life tends to be significantly worse. A survey carried out by researchers from the University of California, San Francisco, of over 13,000 adults aged between twenty and seventy-five revealed that more than half reported acute or chronic pain at levels similar to those reported by people living with terminal cancer. And almost a quarter reported fatigue, depression, sleep disturbance and physical and emotional disability. These symptoms were present across the entire course of the disease, spanning all age ranges but with increasing prevalence towards the end of life.[1]

Many of these symptoms may also be a result of the side effects of the drugs prescribed for treatment. It's acknowledged that higher average blood glucose levels (measured by HbA1C) are associated with a greater risk that there will be complications of the disease. The conventional medical model has revolved around keeping this under control with the use of medication. In those with type-1 diabetes (an autoimmune condition in which the pancreas stops producing insulin), these drugs are life-saving. Type-1 is not related to lifestyle, whereas in type-2 diabetes, which is almost entirely preventable, glucose-lowering medications do not prolong life, or reduce stroke rates or death rates from heart disease. What makes it worse is that the side effects from these medications are responsible for 100,000 visits to the Emergency Room (ER) every year in the US.[2]

In the UK, the cost of insulin and oral diabetes medications has increased by over 300 per cent in the past few years and the combined cost to the NHS has now reached in excess of £700 million per annum.[3]

Think about that for a second. We spend hundreds of millions of taxpayers' money on diabetes drugs, yet they do not have any impact on preventing some of the most important adverse health outcomes for patients with type-2 diabetes. In 2014, I, Dr Ben Maruthappu, a senior doctor working under the CEO of the NHS (Simon Stevens), and the chair of the Academy of Medical Royal Colleges, Professor Terence Stephenson (now chairman of the General Medical Council), wrote in a medical journal editorial that doctors should be clear about what the limited marginal benefits of these drugs are in combination and they should also inform patients about the impact of a Mediterranean diet, which would have a much greater effect on a patient's health and be free from side effects.[4]

Instead, many patients believe that the advice is to follow a low-fat, high-carbohydrate diet in order to prevent heart disease, and that the dosage of drugs will be adjusted accordingly. Take, for example, the man who called into a national radio show in Cape Town, South Africa, on which I was a guest to discuss the relationship between diet and heart disease. Diagnosed with type-2 diabetes, he was under the impression that he had to consume sugar in order for his diabetes medications to 'work' – when in fact his sugar intake was only making him worse.

It is estimated that there are currently 3.1 million people living with type-2 diabetes in the UK; it is the single greatest cost to the NHS; and its prevalence has more than doubled in the last twenty years.

When one factors in the added cost of lost productivity due to sickness, type-2 diabetes is costing the UK £20 billion per annum. Without significant steps being taken to reduce the number of sufferers, it is estimated that this figure will reach a colossal £40 billion by 2035. In the US, the total cost of diabetes reached $245 billion by 2012, a 40 per cent increase in just five years.

Type-2 diabetes is certainly a condition to avoid if you can, but it's not all doom and gloom. There's a substantial body of scientific evidence that reveals that the condition can be reversed or, at the very least, that sufferers will be able to come off medication if they make changes to their diet. This goes against what I was taught at medical school, which is that type-2 diabetes is a 'chronic irreversible condition'. The most extensive piece of research to date looking at all available evidence was a paper, 'Dietary Carbohydrate Restriction as the First Approach in Diabetes Management: Critical Review and Evidence Base', published in *Nutrition and Metabolism* in 2015. It outlined research led by pioneering biochemist Dr Richard Feinman and including twenty-six international leaders in the fields of biochemistry, medicine, nutrition and obesity.[5]

Their conclusions were summarized in twelve points:

1. Hyperglycaemia is the most salient feature of diabetes. Dietary carbohydrate restriction has the greatest effect on decreasing blood glucose levels.

2. During the epidemics of obesity and type 2 diabetes, caloric increases have been due almost entirely to increased carbohydrates.

3. Benefits of dietary carbohydrate restriction do not require weight loss.

4. Although weight loss is not required for benefit, no dietary intervention is better than carbohydrate restriction for weight loss.

5. Adherence to low-carbohydrate diets in people with type-2 diabetes is at least as good as adherence to any other dietary interventions and is frequently significantly better.

6. Replacement of carbohydrates with protein is generally beneficial.

7. Dietary total and saturated fat do not correlate with risk for cardiovascular disease.

8. Plasma saturated fatty acids are controlled by dietary carbohydrates more than dietary lipids.

9. The best predictor of microvascular complications and, to a lesser extent, macrovascular complications is glycaemic control.

10. Dietary carbohydrate restriction is the most effective method (other than starvation) for reducing serum triglycerides and increasing high-density lipoprotein (HDL).

11. Patients on carbohydrate-restricted diets reduce and frequently eliminate medication. People with type-1 diabetes usually require lower insulin.

12. Intensive glucose lowering through dietary carbohydrate restriction has no side effects, comparable to the effects of intensive pharmacological treatment.

National Diabetes champion GP Dr David Unwin saved close to £40,000 in his own practice on medications for type-2 diabetes in comparison to other practices in his clinical commissioning group, purely by giving simple dietary advice to his patients to cut out the refined carbo-hydrates. If all GPs across the 9,400 practices in the UK gave out this free advice, it could potentially save the NHS £370 million on drugs alone.

Dr Unwin says, 'Telling a patient with diabetes to consume sugar in moderation is moderately poisoning them,' and he's right. However, in effect, all carbohydrates turn into glucose when digested – it's the dose and in what form of food it's consumed that's crucial. Like myself, David is a founding member of the Public Health Collaboration, a not-for-profit charity independent of food-industry interests. The table below gives examples of the effects of many commonly consumed foods translated into teaspoons of sugar according to glucose content.

Food	Serving size (g)	Teaspoons of sugar
Basmati rice, boiled	150	10.1
Potato, white, baked	150	8.2
French fries, baked	150	7.5
Sweetcorn, boiled	80	7.3
Spaghetti, white, boiled	180	6.6
Wholemeal bread, 2 small slices	60	6
Banana, raw	120	5.7
Apple, raw	120	2.3
Frozen peas, boiled	80	1.3
Broccoli, boiled	80	0.2
Eggs	60	0

The consumption of many of these food produces a rapid glucose and insulin spike, and there are very few nutrients in them. I personally don't include bread, pasta or rice as a part of my healthy diet any longer, but see them as occasional treats to eat in small doses.

A programme following the same principles has been set up by another organization, Diabetes.co.uk, independent (i.e. they do not receive any funding or sponsorship) of food and pharmaceutical industry interests. Within just one year, data concluded that the participation of 7,297 type-2 diabetic patients in their low-refined-carbohydrate programme generated a cost saving through reduction in medication of £6.9 million. Extrapolate this across the UK population suffering with type-2 diabetes, and we could save hundreds of millions in the use of medication alone.

In Pioppi, we learned that pasta was never a main course but was always eaten as a starter. Interestingly, when you add extra virgin olive oil to bread or pasta, its glycaemic index is reduced; in other words, the glucose and insulin response in the bloodstream isn't so marked. Vinegar, which is also a popular staple in Mediterranean regions, has been shown to increase insulin sensitivity in type-2 diabetes patients by more than 30 per cent.

And what about pizza in Pioppi? Well, they eat it only once or twice a month. The combination of all the positives in their diet and lifestyle, and a refined-sugar consumption of virtually zero, makes it easy to understand why the smaller portions of refined carbohydrate, including freshly baked bread and pizza, consumed don't do them any harm.

In summary:

- Type-2 diabetes is a condition related to the body's inability to metabolize carbohydrates

- It's a multi-organ condition characterized by raised blood glucose that increases the risk of heart attack, stroke, peripheral vascular disease, eye disease, kidney disease and nerve damage

- The condition can be managed and potentially reversed from following a diet low in refined carbohydrates

- Benefits from carbohydrate restriction are independent of weight loss

- In Pioppi, pasta is never eaten as a main course and pizza is consumed only once or twice a month

9.

Stop Counting Calories and Stop Snacking

'It's extremely naïve of the public and the medical profession to think that a calorie of bread, a calorie of meat and a calorie of alcohol have the same metabolic effects on the body.'

– Professor David Haslam, Chairman,
National Obesity Forum

For decades, the public health message has been that 'a calorie is a calorie is a calorie' and that all calories count, no matter where they come from. As a result of this fictitious message becoming conventional wisdom, the food industry has profited from the successful promotion of low-calorie processed foods and these have been harmful to the public's health. What does the science really tell us?

When it comes to physics, a calorie is a measure of energy. Fat has nine calories per gram, and both protein and carbohydrate have four calories per gram. But when we look at biochemistry – essentially, how our body processes, metabolizes and reacts to what we put in our mouths – it's a completely different story: it depends much more on where those calories come from.

As we've seen, fat has the least impact on blood glucose and insulin responses when compared to protein and carbohydrate, but particular types of fat will have a different impact on your health. For example, calories from trans fats will increase your risk of a heart attack, whereas calories from omega-3 fatty acids will protect you from one.

Fibrous carbohydrates from whole fruit and vegetables will be good for your gut and delay the absorption of glucose, whereas the starch in refined carbohydrates like bread, pasta and rice will be rapidly broken down and cause a significantly greater spike in both glucose and insulin. And when it comes to protein, the body has to put in twice as much energy to break it down (the thermic effect of food) compared to carbohydrate.

Other reasons why calorie-focused thinking has been damaging is because it does not address the question of what is good nutrition and it fails to take into consideration the metabolic effect on the body and how different sources of calories affect appetite control. When you intertwine all this with the impact of specific macronutrients on appetite, it's easier to understand why our grandparents didn't count calories and there was very little obesity. The residents of Pioppi were certainly not counting calories – and this is because they are eating nutritious, healthy food and don't snack. When it comes to satiety (feeling full), fat, fibre and protein are kings, while sugar and refined carbohydrates are going to mean that you are constantly feeling hungry.

Until I cut out all sugar and refined carbohydrates from my diet, I thought feeling hungry every couple of hours was normal. On a typical day, I would have a sugared cereal for breakfast and a glass of orange juice, then top off thirty to forty-five minutes in the gym with a 'sports' drink. At work in the hospital, I'd feel hungry again at about 10.30 a.m., so I'd indulge in a KitKat, which would keep me going until 12.30 p.m., when I'd be starving again. My usual lunch was either a pasta dish or a panini and a packet of crisps. About an hour and a half later, after starting to feel lethargic, I'd pop over to the local coffee shop and order a mocha with extra chocolate syrup. Dinner would almost always be a curry and a full plate of rice. And, before bed, I'd crave something sweet, and eat a slice of chocolate cake. The next morning, I'd wake up starving, and the cycle would continue.

However, once I had researched the science and cut added sugar and refined carbs from my diet, I could go for hours without feeling hungry and I found it easy to stop snacking on processed food. Within weeks, I lost around a stone of fat around my waist, without even trying, and my cholesterol profile is now better than ever.

The diagram below explains the effect a constant cycle of eating non-fibrous carbohydrates, such as bread, pasta and rice, has on glucose and insulin.

One of the earliest obesity experiments was carried

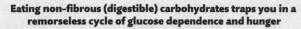

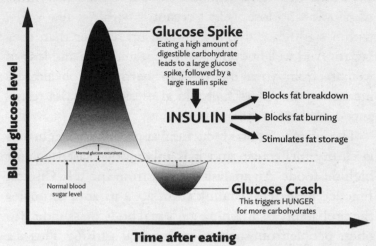

Credit: Dr Ted Naiman

out by researchers A. Kekwick and G. L. Pawan and published in the *Lancet* in 1956. They set up three different groups, one on a diet of 90 per cent fat, one of 90 per cent protein and one of 90 per cent carbohydrate. The number of total calories consumed was the same across all three groups. The greatest weight loss occurred in the fat-consuming group and the authors concluded that 'the composition of the diet appeared to outweigh in importance the intake of calories'.[1]

Scientific evidence clearly reveals that, for people who are overweight or obese, low-fat, low-calorie diets have not only been an epic failure but also potentially harmful. The weight-loss industry, which emphasizes calorie restriction over good nutrition, generates $58 billion annually in the US, despite the fact that more than two thirds of people who lose weight regain it within a few years, with a significant number ending up heavier than they began. And weight cycling (the repeated gain and loss of weight) from yoyo dieting can harm your health by increasing the risk of high blood pressure, insulin resistance and chronic inflammation.[2]

The current 'calorie reduction' approach to weight loss is clearly ineffective, and it is inherently biased against high-fat foods. An analysis of data from the UK Clinical Practice Research Datalink from 2004 to 2014 estimates the probability of attaining a normal body mass index for obese people from such an approach at 1 in 167. This is a failure rate of more than 99 per cent, and the majority of this percentage comes from reduced-calorie diets. Not surprisingly, the authors state, 'Even when treatment is accessed, evidence suggests behavioural weight loss interventions focussing on caloric restriction and increased physical activity are unlikely to yield clinically significant reductions in body weight.'[3]

Look AHEAD (Action for Health in Diabetes) was the largest and longest-lasting randomized controlled trial to see whether health outcomes would improve if participants adopted a calorie-restricted, low-fat diet and increased the amount of exercise they did. The trial looked at over 5,000 overweight or obese patients with type-2 diabetes, but was stopped after ten years. It had proved futile: although the participants who adopted the diet and exercise regime did lose more weight than those in the control group, there was no reduction in the rate of death, heart attacks, stroke or in hospital admissions.[4]

As the PREDIMED trial demonstrated, if the diet had been a high-fat Mediterranean one with no restriction on calories, it's likely that heart attacks, strokes or deaths would have been prevented, and, combining this with further restriction in the consumption of refined carbohydrates, it's highly likely that many patients would have been able to come off medication and potentially reverse the progression of their type-2 diabetes.

The other issue with 'low fat' being seen as synonymous with 'low calorie' is the adverse effect it has on the good cholesterol, HDL, which, as we have seen, after insulin resistance, is the most important element in the prediction of heart attack. Sugar and refined carbohydrates reduce HDL, whereas replacing these foods with fat in the diet from specific foods such as extra virgin olive oil, walnuts, full-fat dairy and coconut oil increases HDL and leads to a drop in triglycerides, which creates an overall improvement in an individual's cholesterol profile.

Another major change that has occurred since the 1970s, when the low-fat diet revolution was embraced, is an increase in the frequency of meals. Prior to 1970 and the obesity epidemic, people generally ate three meals a day: breakfast, lunch and dinner. Fast-forward to the present day, and some of us are now (as I used to) eating six times a day: breakfast, snack, lunch, snack, dinner, snack. And each of these, more often than not, contains sugar. If we are eating continually, from the moment we get up to the moment we go to sleep, our body does not have enough time to digest and use some of the foods that we eat. The entire day becomes an opportunity to store food energy without there being a chance to burn it.

Snacks tend to be highly insulinogenic (or fattening) because we demand the convenience and long shelf life of refined carbohydrates. It is simple to eat some crackers as a snack, more of an effort to eat a small piece of grilled salmon. And it's also likely that the types of snacks we eat, in addition to main meals consisting of processed food, perpetuate a cycle of feeling continuously hungry, and thus our overall unhealthy-calorie consumption increases substantially.

A joint report undertaken by the UK's National Obesity Forum and the Public Health Collaboration, which I co-authored, states, 'Shifting focus away from calories and emphasizing a dietary pattern that focuses on food quality rather than quantity will help to rapidly reduce obesity, related diseases and cardiovascular risk.'

So, Grandma was right: just eat real food and stop snacking, and if you do have to eat the odd snack, make it a healthy one, like a handful of nuts!

In summary:

- Different sources of calories have a different metabolic effect on the body

- When it comes to satiety (feeling full), fat, fibre and protein are kings, but sugar and refined carbohydrates keep you constantly hungry

- Low-fat, calorie-restricted diets do not improve health outcomes

- Low-fat, low-calorie diets have an adverse effect on **HDL** cholesterol

- Weight cycling from yoyo dieting can harm health by increasing the risk of high blood pressure, insulin resistance and chronic inflammation

10.

The Physical Activity Obesity Myth: You Can't Outrun a Bad Diet

'An obese person doesn't have to increase their physical activity level one iota in order to lose weight, they just need to eat less.'

— Lord Ian McColl of Dulwich, Professor of Surgery and former Shadow Health Minister

To say that I have been obsessed with regular exercise is an understatement. I've naturally always been very active from a young age, and I captained sports teams at school and at local club level, winning competitions and trophies in badminton and cricket during my teenage years. I was a leg spin bowler and opening batsman for Manchester Grammar School and, after being selected into the Lancashire County Cricket Club centre of excellence aged sixteen, I had to decide between pursuing a sporting career or following one in medicine. I chose medicine.

The point I'm making is that I have an inherent bias

towards sport and being active. For me, it was predominantly the enjoyment I gained from playing team sports and not initially for the purposes of health.

I've never been overweight by the conventional definition of body mass index but, from my teenage years onwards, I've always carried fat around my belly, which I felt was disproportionate, as I am otherwise slim. I accepted this as a normal part of my genetic make-up, as my father, who has also been very active all his life, also has a pot belly. However, when I cut out the vast quantities of sugar, bread and pasta I had been consuming from my diet, I managed to lose a stone in weight, all, it seemed, from my midriff, without increasing the amount of exercise I was doing. During the making of his first movie, *Cereal Killers*, Donal lost weight despite doing only eight minutes of exercise a week.

Ever since the obesity epidemic became a public health crisis, the conventional wisdom has been that lack of exercise is to blame – in essence, that we're doing less activity and, as a result, we're getting fatter. But this is pure fiction, and has been promulgated, mainly by the food industry, and scientists who received research funding from them, to deflect blame from their irresponsible and aggressive marketing of junk food to the most vulnerable members of society, including children. The food industry has even ingeniously managed to associate processed fast food with sport. In the summer of 2012, I presented a report for BBC *Newsnight* in which I said that, in the midst of an obesity epidemic, it was obscene that we had allowed the main sponsors of the London

Olympics to be companies that sold junk food. Giving companies such as McDonald's and Coca-Cola the most effective marketing platform in the world to promote their brand to billions across the globe perpetuates the message that you can eat what you like as long as you exercise – when nothing could be further from the truth.

In a 2016 article in the *Telegraph*, former Shadow Health Minister and decorated Professor of Surgery Lord Ian McColl wrote, in his analysis of who is to blame for the 'fatness epidemic', 'The culprits are the morally corrupt scientists and politicians who allowed themselves to be manipulated by food suppliers into saying that obesity was due to lack of exercise. They wrongly advocated a low-fat, high-carbohydrate and high-sugar diet which greatly increased the profits of the food industry.' And he was absolutely correct.

So what does the independent science tell us?

Firstly, contrary to popular belief, as obesity has rocketed in the past four decades, there's been very little change in activity levels in the western world.[1] In fact, while there's evidence from several states in the US that average exercise levels may have increased, in the same states, obesity has increased simultaneously.

How can this be explained in terms of the individual?

For many people, exercise can be a very powerful stimulator of appetite. One randomized controlled trial published in the *New England Journal of Medicine* revealed that obese individuals who dieted without exercising lost more weight within a year than those who both dieted and exercised.[2]

Even if one accepts the incorrect notion that 'a calorie is a calorie is a calorie', you get very little return for your investment in exercise when it comes to weight loss. You'd have to walk for forty-five minutes to burn off the calories you consume by eating three biscuits, or run several miles to burn off a burger and chips washed down with a sugary drink.

In reality, 60–75 per cent of the calories you burn are used up by doing absolutely nothing. Even at rest, the body expends considerable energy simply to allow your organs to keep you alive, for example by breathing, maintaining the heart's ability to pump blood around the body and the growth and repair of cells. Keeping this in mind, wouldn't you rather those functions were fuelled by nutritious food as opposed to processed junk?

Patients often tell me that, due to an injury, arthritis or something else that results in them not being able to exercise, they find their weight has increased. This serves to perpetuate the no-exercise-leads-to-obesity myth in their mind. However, on further questioning, I always discover that their diet is one which is high in refined carbohydrates. Professor Tim Noakes says, 'The benefits of exercise are unbelievable, but if you have to exercise to keep your weight down, your diet is wrong.'

Tim developed type-2 diabetes in middle age; he had run seventy marathons. In *Cereal Killers*, Professor Noakes is seen tearing pages out of a book he wrote himself, *The Lore of Running*, which is considered to be the bible for marathon runners. That section he ripped out advised endurance athletes to load up on carbohydrates before a big race, something Tim had been doing for decades. He now realizes this was wrong and harmful. In fact, Tim, who had been involved in sports science research from a very young age, told us during the making of *The Big Fat Fix* that, although he didn't realize the significance at the time, at the age of twenty-eight his fasting blood insulin was forty – four times what is now considered the normal upper limit. So, he was insulin resistant decades before he developed type-2 diabetes. He has now managed to control this with a low-carbohydrate diet.

Am I saying all this to diminish the importance of exercise? Of course not. In a report I co-authored and edited for the Academy of Medical Royal Colleges entitled 'Exercise: The Miracle Cure', we made it clear that regular physical activity has many benefits in reducing an individual's risk of developing many chronic diseases, such as heart disease, type-2 diabetes, dementia and some cancers by at least 30 per cent.[3]

It's simply that weight loss is not one of them. It's what you put in your mouth that's rather more important.

However, exercising in the correct way and thus reducing the risk of injury is also crucial. Engaging in 'mindful movement' is perhaps a better description of what we should all be thinking about. (Donal discusses this in more detail in Chapters 11 and 12.) For most people, running on the road or a hard surface can be detrimental for the joints. Every single orthopaedic surgeon I've spoken to says the same thing: no one should be running on the road. Many have operated on patients who have needed a knee or hip replacement in their thirties or forties after years of pounding their joints on a hard surface. Having myself suffered from chronic pain in my knees after a decade of running 15km a week, I've completely changed my own cardio training to daily brisk walking for thirty minutes, interspersed with High Intensity Interval Training (HIIT) for four minutes three times a week. There's also good evidence to suggest that walking may protect against heart disease more effectively than does running. Getting at least 150 minutes of moderate activity a week (twenty-two minutes of brisk walking a day) can add up to four and a half years to life expectancy, independent of body weight.[4]

As I've pointed out, there's no such thing as a healthy weight, and it's imperative that regular physical activity be prescribed for everyone, of all shapes and sizes, including those with a normal body mass index. Public-health messaging must stop using obesity as a reason to encourage the population to keep active.

There also appear to be health benefits to be gained from the activity of having regular sex. A study published in the *American Journal of Cardiology* looked at over a thousand men in their fifties, initially free of cardiovascular disease and followed up for sixteen years, and found that those who had sex only once a month, compared to those having intercourse at least twice a week, were 45 per cent more likely to develop cardiovascular disease during the period studied. One of the researchers noted that those who were having more sex may also be more likely to be those in close or intimate, supportive relationships, and that this in itself may be good for health by reducing stress.[5]

So, what's the most important message? To sum up: keep moving for health reasons, not in order to lose weight, and do something you enjoy, whether it's dancing, cycling, sex or all three – but perhaps not at the same time!

In summary:

- The body burns 60 to 75 per cent of calories when no physical activity is being done, to keep the organs and cells functioning

- There's been very little change in average levels of activity as obesity has rocketed in the past four decades

- Exercise has many benefits, but weight loss is not one of them

- Walking may be more effective than running in preventing heart disease

- Regular sex is good for the heart

11.

Movement is Medicine

'"Did the people here traditionally
engage in any exercise?"
Laughs. "No."'

– Susan Bessie Haslam in an interview for
The Big Fat Fix at the Museum of the
Mediterranean Diet, Pioppi

The Pioppi Paradox? Let's take a closer look . . .

In 1968 Dr Ken Cooper laid the foundations for the
aerobics and jogging boom that was to be with us throughout the 1970s and 1980s. Dr Cooper's points-based system
centred on aerobic, endurance-based physical activity as
the key to better cardiovascular and whole-body health.

During his career with the US Air Force, Dr Cooper
had used a simple twelve-minute running-for-distance test
to establish the fitness of military men and women. From
the result of each 'Cooper Test', he derived a reasonable
estimate of the participant's V_{O2} Max (the gold standard
for cardiovascular fitness) by using the following formula:
(Distance in metres covered in 12 minutes − 504.9/44.73.

In a later publication, he would refine the test to become a 1.5-mile run against the clock. Many police and military regimes continue to use an interpretation of the original Cooper Test today and government recommendations to walk 10,000 steps daily can be directly attributed to Cooper's original work.

Observational studies are supportive, indicating that Vo2 Max – which can be increased by exercise – is indeed a strong predictor of longevity. One such study of Tour de France competitors (who had competed in 1930–64) found that the average age to which the cyclists lived was eighty-one; the non-cyclists in the study on average lived to seventy-three.[1]

If this is indeed compelling and consistent with the science, before you get on your bike you might be interested to know that the average male in Pioppi outlives those elite cyclists by an additional eight years. That he does so with no evidence of scheduled exercise – ever – just seems odd, doesn't it? Although several new gyms were either planned or under construction when we visited the area, such facilities have come about eighty years too late to have had any influence the longevity of the local centenarians!

So, if you can live to eighty-nine without exercise, that obviously begs the question: is exercise really that important after all?

Part of the answer probably lies somewhere in the fields the villagers in Pioppi traditionally worked and the results of a Danish study that indicated that 'the relative intensity, and not the duration of cycling, is of more importance in relation to all-cause and coronary heart disease mortality'.[2]

In the study, men who engaged in fast-intensity cycling survived 5.3 years longer, and men who cycled with average intensity 2.9 years longer, than men who had slow cycling intensity. For women, the figures were 3.9 and 2.2 years longer, respectively. In that context, if we consider the format of the daily 'work' in the fields which the men of Pioppi engaged in habitually throughout their adult life, we would find evidence of varying intensities. They would have easily surpassed the current recommendations of 10,000 steps a day and satisfied those recommendations for higher-intensity efforts with intermittent wood chopping and other more physically demanding tasks.

Exercise as we know it was not important because these men were on the move and putting their bodies to work – consistently so – in the course of their daily activities. As Mayor Pisani explained when we interviewed him for *The Big Fat Fix*, that 'work' is very much identified as a key component of the Mediterranean *diaita* in its original context. Just like the imposed periods of food restriction and fasting, physical activity was a very simple, unconscious fact of life in the region. There was simply no option to outsource movement to automobiles and farm machinery, or food supply to third-party producers. Life was an 'all for one' community effort with bartering of vegetables for fish, fish for wine and olive oil for all.

If such communion of spirit is difficult to replicate in a modern urban environment, can we at least emulate the health benefits of that 'work' component of the *diaita*? And if so, is exercise the best and/or the only answer?

The reality is that, until the 1970s, scheduled exercise was pretty much non-existent outside of team sports, yet the global population was much leaner than it is today. For example, just 127 runners entered the first New York City marathon in 1970 but, as Dr Cooper's philosophy gained traction, endurance exercise bulldozed its way into the public consciousness. With Nike and Jane Fonda leading from the front, simple movement was left behind.

Until that point, exercise had really been a subset of movement – something everyone engaged in before cars and corner couches took over – but that was all about to change. The emergence of jogging, Jane and marathons coincided perfectly with the concept of calories in and calories out (CICO) as the governing law for losing or gaining weight, or maintaining one's ideal weight. That 98,247 runners have applied for the available 50,000 places in the 2017 New York City marathon is a clear indication of how compelling that narrative has been ever since.

It was simple, easy to follow, and the logic behind it very much believable. What could possibly go wrong? Well, quite a lot.

Aseem's 2015 paper in the *British Journal of Sports Medicine*, 'It's Time to Bust the Myth of Physical Activity and Obesity – You Cannot Outrun a Bad Diet', firmly sets out the case against this misguided concept.

One of his co-authors on that paper, the world's leading endurance sports scientist, Professor Tim Noakes, agrees that exercise has many benefits but says that weight loss is not one of them. Interestingly, it was also Noakes who, at the outset of a remarkable career, successfully dismantled the conviction that running marathons eradicated one's risk of heart disease (a story very well told in his autobiography, *Challenging Beliefs*). If we focus exclusively on the benefits Noakes alludes to, the next question is clearly how best to access them if you're not working in the fields of the Mediterranean with the sun on your back every day for the duration of your adult working life.

The most robust research for exercise as an anti-ageing protocol points to the power of higher-intensity interval training protocols (HIIT). Many studies have demonstrated the ability of well-formulated HIIT programmes to mimic and match the aerobic and cardiovascular fitness gains of endurance exercise in just 10 per cent of the time allocated to 'active effort'. In Professor Izumi Tabata's groundbreaking 1990s work, this amounted to four minutes of high-intensity effort (twenty seconds of maximal effort – on a stationary bike, for example – followed by ten seconds' rest, repeated eight times) rather than forty minutes of steady-state endurance training. When you then consider the superior anaerobic (think strength, speed and power) gains of HIIT over steady-state endurance protocols, the case for efficacy is pretty much closed. If you are going to exercise for health benefits, why not do so as smartly and time efficiently as possible?

If good movement is the foundation of safe exercise, then HIIT is the secret sauce of the exercise world. Everyone loves (to hate?) it, because the science behind it being a beneficial intervention is simply rock solid, whatever your base level of fitness. Even if your mobility is poor or impaired, there is always a way to do the programme – for example, open a door, then grab a handle on either side for bodyweight squats, keeping your arms straight and acting as levers. This 'closed chain' supports your structure and protects you from injury, but it still enables you to hit the muscles that matter most with a safe squatting movement.

I was a track and field athlete, and there are many good reasons why interval training was a core part of my own training protocol, as it remains for any elite athlete today. Back then, that's what we called it – interval training; we certainly didn't need the 'high intensity' prefix to assure us that the coach meant business! Fartlek training was another constant in our programme. That was a thirty- to forty-minute run at a slow pace with a short, sharp set of jumping exercises to be completed every minute or so. My middle-distance peers would do a very similar session by running slowly for several minutes' recovery between race-pace repeats of 800 to 1,000 metres. I made the mistake of joining a four-minute-miler for one such session. After hanging on to his coat tails for the first kilometre, I needed a set of binoculars for the next few. It hurt, it worked and athletes have been doing it religiously, long before the great Roger Bannister used an interval-training protocol to break the four-minute mile in 1954. Bannister had time constraints, as he was studying to be a doctor, so the training he did was fast, intense and typically less than forty-five minutes in duration. That he successfully qualified as a doctor just six weeks after his record-breaking run is perhaps the greatest demonstration of the efficacy of interval training.

Fortunately, we don't have to aim for world records or to run a mile in under four minutes reap the benefits. You can even start with interval walking. Recent research has demonstrated that walking at a varied pace is significantly more effective than one-pace walking, even when average speed and distance covered is equal.

In *The Big Fat Fix*, I take Aseem through one of my very simple 'go to' fitness tests – the 300, so-called because it is simply a hundred repetitions of three distinct body-weight exercises. On camera, he compares it to his standard 5km treadmill run in the gym: '*Much* harder!'

As true as that may be, it also takes less than half the time, and it offers up those added benefits we referred to earlier. When I first started to experiment with HIIT in isolation (I had always done it as an athlete, but as part of a much broader training programme) about ten years ago, I set myself the challenge of trying to improve my best time on a particular running route – without running for six weeks.

My N=1 protocol consisted exclusively of high-intensity full-body exercises (lots of old-fashioned, devastatingly effective burpees!) with no one session lasting more than ten minutes. I prioritized the major muscle groups, hitting the gluteus maximus – the largest and most powerful muscle in the body – hard in a bid to improve speed and power, relying on the science, which indicated that aerobic gains were a given with such an approach.

The results were impressive. After six weeks of no

running but exclusively doing full-body HIIT training for a total of no more than thirty minutes a week, I broke ten minutes on my first outing. I had just knocked sixteen seconds off my previous best effort – and taught myself a valuable lesson.

In hindsight, I probably learned more in those six weeks than I had done throughout my competitive career at an incomparably elite level. My body loves to run, but my bad back sometimes doesn't, so, initially, I was simply trying to navigate my way around that challenge. How to stay strong and mobile as our body changes over time is something we must all face in our own way, and the Twenty-one-day Movement Protocol is designed to help you do just that.

If HIIT training really does seem to be the gift that keeps on giving, it nonetheless suffers from serial abuse in a very commercial multibillion-dollar exercise industry. When you consider that recent research in Canada demonstrated that a once-weekly set of twenty-second maximal efforts three times with a few minutes for recovery between each rep serves up remarkable benefits, it pains me to see folks attempt to 'do more' because that doesn't feel like it's enough.

Enough for what?

If you overdo the volume of exercise, you will be working against the benefits of HIIT, which requires maximum effort for very short periods of time; and once you reduce the effort in order to keep going for longer, you defeat the purpose – and dilute the benefits – instantaneously. I always think of HIIT as the espresso of exercise: short, strong and slightly bitter, but damned effective.

I was not at all surprised that my 'eight minute per week' exercise protocol in *Cereal Killers* was mocked for its brevity and simplicity. As with food, many folks presume themselves to be knowledgeable to the point of expertise about exercise simply because they have been eating every day for forty years or exercising regularly! Unfortunately, this is not the case.

Competitive athletes know this intuitively, of course. They and their coaches operate from a place of specificity, focusing explicitly on improving performance in their given sporting discipline. I know of one world-record holder from my own era for whom a complete training session was five thirty-metre sprints with fifteen minutes' full recovery between each one. That may sound like very little but, as a sprint athlete, he was 100 per cent focused on improving speed, so in fact it makes complete sense. The long-distance athlete may complete ten or fifteen 400-metre runs – same principle, but a different set-up. What all elite coaches do is marry the very best available scientific research with the wisdom of their own experience and an intuitive knowledge of each athlete. As a framework, that makes complete sense.

When we view healthy ageing through a similar prism – where the 'performance' challenges we face are a very different kettle of fish – it bemuses me to see that so many of us choose to ignore the irrefutable evidence of what in reality works best and to opt for what we think we know best.

For those ageing people who do choose to exercise, endurance training tends to be the default option, but it simply cannot compete as an anti-ageing intervention when compared to HIIT protocols. Don't get me wrong, it is still a *great* thing to do, it's just not the *best* thing you can do as you become older.

In fact, if we consider the jaw-dropping findings of one very recent study by the Mayo Clinic in the US, it seems reasonable to suggest that short, sharp bursts of exercise are like kryptonite to the ageing process. That study showed that HIIT 'robustly improved cardio-respiratory fitness, insulin sensitivity, mitochondrial respiration, and fat-free mass (FFM)', all of which are key processes diluted by the ageing process. They saw a whopping 69 per cent increase in 'the ability of the mitochondria within cells to generate energy in older subjects'. In that context, the eight-minute weekly exercise protocol I structured for *Cereal Killers* no longer looks so crazy. That's also why I put Aseem through his paces in *The Big Fat Fix* in similar fashion, and why I would encourage you to give HIIT – as laid out in the Twenty-one-day Movement Protocol – a try.

Still not convinced? Then these MRI scans of three people's thighs showing the benefits of quality exercise over time are a compelling visual of how we can maintain – or lose – lean muscle as we age. Use it or lose it? You bet![3]

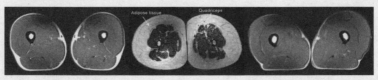

40 year-old triathlete   74 year-old sedentary   70 year-old triathlete

But before you do that . . .

When I feel great these days, I sprint, but 90 per cent of my time spent moving is dedicated to nurturing mobility, and I would encourage you to think along similar lines. Learn to move well before you move fast or attempt to lift anything other than your own body weight!

It may surprise you, but it is within this context that I would demote exercise to second place behind habitual, constant daily movement – like that engaged in by the people of Pioppi. There is one very simple but compelling reason for this. We are sitting too much these days, and the case for sedentary behaviour being a negative health option is growing ever stronger.

When we swapped movement for exercise back in the 1970s, the simple CICO equation suggested that sitting at a desk for eight hours each day wouldn't have a negative impact on our health and fitness if we were working out, feeling the burn and hitting our calorie-expenditure target for the day.

Unfortunately, the reality is somewhat different.

Sedentary time has now been independently linked to poor health outcomes – and that's irrespective of time spent exercising. As we explain more fully in Chapter 12, telomeres, a key indicator of ageing, are a region of repetitive DNA at the end of a chromosome which protects the end of the chromosome from deterioration. One recent study found that telomere lengthening was 'significantly associated with reduced sitting time'.[4]

Of course, if 'not sitting' is in itself a positive health decision, the recent trend towards 'standing' desks might seem to make sense. But hold on a moment. The research points more towards the power of movement than simply to swapping our sedentary sitting for sedentary standing. What does seem to do the trick is a two- to three-minute movement break every forty-five minutes.

Is that too much to ask?

Within two minutes of standing up, your body responds positively at a cellular level, rewarding you richly for a simple decision to move around a little. From a scientific perspective, we are not entirely sure why this is the case, but sometimes we don't need science to confirm what we know and feel in our DNA.

The 206 bones, 650 skeletal muscles and that complex cardiovascular system we each call our own are superbly designed to host, nurture and enjoy habitual movement. Man was made to move!

In *The Big Fat Fix*, our director of human movement (a first such role for any movie!), Louise, takes Aseem through a process of realignment. His body was showing visible signs of too much sitting but, with Louise's guidance, he found his way back to a much more balanced alignment relatively quickly – something the before-and-after shots demonstrate very clearly. There are some very simple ways to guide yourself to good alignment. Louise speaks about aligning the head over the heart centre/ribcage, and over the pelvis, over the full length of the feet. Once you align these parts, the mechanics are on your side and you can progress safely to the more advanced movement and resistance training challenges you see us undertaking in the movie.

Learn to move better, then start to move more!

Whatever your starting point, the remarkable ability of the body to recover its form and find its way back to baseline health never ceases to amaze me. If you give it a chance to guide you accordingly, the body will reward you with improved energy, mobility and health.

Sadly, the fact that immobility correlates very closely indeed with all-cause mortality over a ten-year period is either ignored, forgotten or never fully understood the first instance – and I can assure you that my own experience of immobility, albeit at a young age, was revealing in this context. The back injury I sustained, at the age of just sixteen, while training as an international track and field competitor, ended my sporting career and still resonates today in everything I do.

After several bouts of major surgery, it took me a full fifteen years to find my way back to pain-free mobility. There were days when I could not tie my shoelaces and my only movement was confined to the weight-bearing environment of the swimming pool.

'If your spine is inflexibly stiff at thirty, you are old. If it is completely flexible at sixty, you are young.' So said Joseph Pilates and, believe me, I know exactly what he meant.

Fundamentally, though, I found ways to keep moving and explored ways to move better and to reprogramme my body to function better. Yoga sounded like a viable option, and my first teacher, in Australia, was excellent. Back in Dublin, however, I limped out of my first and only class with severely compromised mobility. I can now do yoga safely only thanks to my immersion in Pilates, t'ai chi and natural movement protocols since then. However you choose to move, never overestimate your ability, and move as safely as possible.

To check in with where you are right now, one of the simplest – but at the same time remarkably revealing – tests of mobility is the Sit-Rise Test (SRT) developed by Brazilian researchers. The SRT requires you to start in a standing position then to sit down on the ground with the least assistance possible, before rising again to a standing position. It is scored out of ten, with one point deducted for every time you touch the ground with a body part other than your feet for assistance. If you use your hand to help you sit down, you lose a point; likewise, if you use a hand and knee to support you on the way back up, two additional points would be taken away, leaving you with a total score of seven.

In a paper published in 2012, the authors concluded that, over a ten-year period, 'Musculoskeletal fitness, as assessed by SRT, was a significant predictor of mortality in 51–80-year-old subjects.'[5]

The paper makes no mention of the fact that the SRT is also an entertaining party piece – something I discovered when presenting it to 300 children in a primary school in Mumbai this year. This simple challenge proved a great opener, and it got their attention, they had some fun and it left them with a positive message of movement. They loved it.

Now that we understand the importance of mobility as we age, the movement elements of the Pioppi Diet are uniquely designed to help you improve your own physical functionality. If you follow them closely, you should find yourself physically prepared to safely up the ante with more demanding HIIT or resistance-training options (should you wish to do so). Importantly, when you walk, try to be mindful of your posture, breathing and surroundings as much as possible.

Of course, if we relate all this to the menfolk of Pioppi, their movement would have been a mixture of walking and working, but, most significantly, it was varied – stop, start, uphill, downhill (the region is very hilly) – and with frequent breaks and shorter bursts of intensity.

That's something to think about: the walking you do need not happen all in one dose and, in fact, you may be even better off spreading it out across your day. So, take those stairs and be alert for opportunities to add more movement to your day – the more varied, the better.

One of the reasons Aseem loves to recommend walking to his patients is that it is freely available, super-effective and open to all. No excuses! As for me, I encourage it because walking with purpose presents a fantastic opportunity to oil the joints, realign your posture and engage with the world around you.

Louise literally put Aseem through his paces in *The Big Fat Fix* to improve his locomotion when walking, and it is a fact that many of us do not use our feet and calf muscles to propel ourselves forward, as we should do. That calf pump Louise refers to is also beneficial to circulation, and it's another reason why I wear only Grandt Mason's Bearthfoot shoes these days. Learn to feel your feet!

Recent research also indicates that moving or walking in nature can improve cognition performance more than in an urban environment, which again points to the power exercised by the environment that we experienced in Pioppi. The Japanese use a term, 'forest bathing', which I like a lot. In practice, it means spending time fully immersed in nature. In this context, you might say that the 'work' in Pioppi was, in effect, a life-long experiment in nature bathing! *La dolce vita*, indeed.

So, find a park, vary your pace and get out there and move. Even if your mobility is compromised by age, injury or pain, every short walk you take is a minor step to major gains. While you're out there, see if you can spot some of the very best examples of posturally correct movement in young children playing.

Until we are seven or eight years old, our movement is perfectly fluid yet entirely unconscious. We move well because it feels good! Dr Laurie Rauch points out that 'correct movement execution feels good because it leads to balanced chemical release, letting us know the movement is executed well'. The children do not know this, of course, but each child's body certainly does.

That innate ability resides in all of us, and by introducing some mindful movement into our day-to-day life, we really can learn to tune in and listen to our body once more.

Taking all this into consideration, I hope you can now see that the absence of gyms and exercise in Pioppi is not a paradox at all. The fact is, movement has been underrated – and exercise overrated – for too long now, and it's high time we recognized and responded to that.

If you learn to move better, and then move more often, these minor changes will help you enjoy significant health gains over time. After that, some smarter HIIT-style or resistance exercise is really just the icing on the cake.

In summary:

- There were no gyms in Pioppi, yet the local men outlive elite Tour de France cyclists by almost a decade – without any scheduled exercise!

- The Pioppi Paradox? No! Mayor Pisani explained that the manual labour these men engaged in daily is an essential part of the original *diaita*

- Being sedentary is an independent risk factor for ill health. Take mini movement breaks – do not sit for more than forty-five minutes at a time

- Moving better and more often, plus some higher-intensity exercises (HIIT), can combat the physical effects of ageing

- Walk where possible, try the SRT Test and start the Twenty-one-day Movement Protocol immediately

12.

Stress

'There's not much sign of stress around here
(Pioppi), Aseem.'

– Donal to Aseem in *The Big Fat Fix*

If many visible signs and clues to longevity revealed themselves to us in our visit to Pioppi – from the siesta to the sunshine, the social connections and the habitual movement – perhaps the most powerful of all was one which we couldn't see at all.

Stress.

We've all felt it, haven't we?

Regardless of your age, marital status, ethnicity, nationality, income or education, the characteristics of a stressful situation are common – and recognizable – to all of us.

While the circumstances that trigger a stress response may differ for each of us, the recipe – and the result – is universal. Specifically, studies have shown that one or more of the 'NUTS' factors must be in play: Novelty, Unpredictability, Threat to the ego, or poor Sense of control.

Sometimes, stress can be a positive force, motivating you

to perform well at a given time, on a critical task at work, for example. But more often than not – for instance when you're sitting in traffic and running late – stress is a negative force.

Your body responds to stress with a perfectly normal, strategic release of a select basket of hormones designed to help us to meet the demands of the prevailing situation. Adrenaline, the 'warrior' hormone, kicks in immediately to help prepare you for a physical response – your heart pumps faster, your breathing rate picks up and more blood starts flowing to your muscles. You are primed for action!

Cortisol, the spy hormone, is next on the scene, about ten minutes later. Acting as a back-up for adrenaline and to maintain those high energy levels, cortisol helps to turn stored fat and carbohydrates into simple fats and sugars we can use as fuel to deal with the acute crisis. It also acts as a natural anti-inflammatory and sharpens our senses before eventually assisting with the physiological 'return to normal' process.

If this ancient 'fight or flight' response served ancestral humans very well in our hunter-gatherer phase, the problem today is that we hunt on the internet and gather by car. Over time, the complete absence of any physical outlet to flush the body of these stress hormones sets the table for negative health outcomes.

You are primed for action . . . but then there is no action!

This type of random stress event is recognizable to all of us, but experiencing stress over a prolonged period of time is much more serious. The multiple challenges we face every day, such as work deadlines, commuter traffic, financial concerns and family issues, can all trigger a stress response. And, although the circumstances that generally trigger stress in the modern environment differ drastically from the life-or-death situations our ancestors experienced, the response is in fact identical.

Without effective tools to manage stress, the aggregation of these multiple stressors can leave you stuck in that fight-or-flight gear. Although beneficial in acute situations, over time this constant state of alert can have serious consequences for your health.

When the body prioritizes survival during an acute stressful event, lots of energy is redirected in response – increased heart rate, elevated blood pressure, increased fuel release into the bloodstream – and it has to go somewhere. Avoiding a predator would definitely have used up this energy, but sitting in your car for an hour after work doesn't have quite the same effect. In a world with reduced movement and activity, our ancient pot of stress hormones can very easily simmer.

You are primed for action . . . but then there is no action . . . so you are still primed for action!

In reality, although you have very probably (grossly) exaggerated the 'danger' confronting you, your perception of that danger will nonetheless trigger the cascade of life-saving hormones, even though you don't actually need them.

So, what happens next?

Although we think of stress as an invisible, psychological predator, this rush of hormones essentially seeps into your body at the very deepest cellular level. If you allow those hormones to stew by continuously ruminating on past (or future) events, the implications can be devastating, up to and including an alteration in your gene expression.

That's probably why we tend to pick up on it quite easily when someone we know is 'carrying the weight of the world' on their shoulders. Suffice to say, there was no evidence of such negative rumination among the people we met in Pioppi!

It is for this reason that Louise encourages us in *The Big Fat Fix* to respond to acute stress situations, such as a run-in with your boss, with movement and activity (if possible): 'Get up, do some squats, get moving!' she says. Doing so will help us mimic the response of our ancestors and flush out the stress hormones, expediting the return to a normal, balanced state of body and mind. In this context, movement really is medicine.

One of the more exciting areas of research that overlaps neatly with this is that into telomeres and telomerase activity. Telomeres are an essential part of human cells and affect how our cells age. Because they 'cap' the end sequences of DNA chromosomes, telomeres are often compared to the plastic tips on shoelaces. In young cells, an enzyme called telomerase rebuilds the end of telomeres and keeps them from wearing down too much but, as we age, the availability of telomerase naturally declines, the telomeres grow shorter and the cells age. This is inevitable for all of us.

Studies exposing human cells to telomerase have slowed cell ageing and even allowed the cells to begin replicating again. Lengthening telomeres has also been shown to have a favourable impact on gene expression, which then prompts cells to behave as though they were younger.

If the mechanisms are complex, the concept of physically measuring part of a chromosome from point A to point B and aligning that with ageing is appealing for many reasons. To most of us, the simplicity of this type of analysis is compelling, and very easy to grasp. You are sixty-four. Your cells are fifty-eight. Well done.

In the science of ageing, length matters and telomeres are sexy as hell.

That being the case, it is clearly in our best interests to maintain cell integrity and telomere length as best we can, for as long as we can. And if telomere maintenance is a long game, the people of Pioppi are ticking many of the boxes we now know matter in this context. Top of that list?

Stress!

Chronic stress was first linked to compromised telomere maintenance in a groundbreaking 2004 study by Nobel laureate Elizabeth Blackburn. Since then, researchers have corroborated those conclusions by consistently demonstrating a link between chronic stress and telomere shortening.

Meanwhile, both telomere shortness and stress have independently been associated with several lifestyle diseases, including heart disease and type-2 diabetes. Although we don't yet fully understand the detailed mechanisms and pathways involved, the totality of the evidence is very clear: chronic stress can be devastating to human health. (In fact, the Pioppi Diet addresses all the known enemies of telomere integrity. In addition to stress, all the following are acknowledged to have a deleterious impact on telomere length: not enough movement, restricted sleep, smoking and poor diet.)

Clearly, on a day-to-day basis, we cannot all be measuring our telomeres, but heart rate variability (HRV) – the interval between your heartbeats – is a useful proxy you could measure relatively easily, using any one of the many free mobile-phone apps out there.

Much more importantly, whether you choose to measure HRV or not, there is much we can do to manage our response to external stressors more effectively.

In *The Big Fat Fix*, Dr Laurie Rauch says that today, 'Going to work is like going to war.' Indeed, if you consider what a traditional lifestyle in Pioppi must have been like, then our modern environment is pretty much a battlefield across the board!

To mimic the low levels of stress we could very much feel during the filming we did in Pioppi is challenging, but not impossible. The critical factor is that your body must not be operating merely as a survival machine and in that constant fight-or-flight mode. This state actively reduces your HRV (a high HRV indicates a healthy, stress-free person) and accelerates telomere shortening, an outcome it is good to avoid.

To successfully manage our response, we need to understand the role that our autonomic nervous system (ANS) plays in all this. The ANS is made up of two 'separate' systems: the ('fight or flight') sympathetic nervous system (SNS), and the ('rest and recovery') parasympathetic nervous system (PSNS).

Maintaining the balance between these two systems is

a key component of general health and healthy ageing. The good news is that your 'rest and recovery' PSNS is even more powerful than the SNS – in the right hands (or head!), that is.

In *The Big Fat Fix*, after Louise had realigned Aseem's body and prepped him for better movement, we used various balance challenges to help Aseem trigger and train his response to an external stressor. When you balance on something, the fear of falling off immediately activates your SNS. The standard response is a defensive 'tightening up', at which point you will lose balance and fall off (the log, in Aseem's case).

In that situation, the only solution available for Aseem to meet the challenge being presented to his body was a physical adjustment; if your centre of gravity is off, the laws of physics determine very quickly that you cannot maintain balance. So, by having Aseem focus on the critical components required to meet his external stressor by means of simple cues – specifically, his posture ('Think of a plumbline through the top of the head'), his breathing ('Let the shoulders relax, breathe slowly'), his weight distribution ('Find your feet') and the alignment of the body in space ('Eyes forward') – he became more proficient at using his PSNS to 'crowd out' his SNS response and successfully navigate the unstable log. Basically, he learned to relax and respond better to a given stimulus.

At one point in the film I make a reference to the great American tennis player Arthur Ashe. He perhaps summed up this process best when he said, 'The ideal attitude is to be physically loose and mentally tight.'

I am too young to remember Arthur Ashe's playing days but, in the modern sporting era, the balletic Roger Federer is surely the greatest example and exponent of this advice. In contrast, some of the most prominent examples of SNS going into destructive overdrive can be seen regularly in the world of sports, where the legacy (and financial) implications can be enormous.

Think of the golfer who misses a very short putt to lose a major title, or the tennis player who chokes in the final set in a Wimbledon final with a series of double faults. How can a trained professional who has served millions of balls successfully suddenly and completely collapse at such a career-defining moment?

Why does an outstanding American Football quarter-back make the worst split-second decision of his career and in so doing lose a Super Bowl in the dying minutes? Why does the English football team consistently lose on penalty shootouts?

In contrast, when we consider that PSNS activation decreases our pulse, breathing rates and blood pressure and then constricts the pupils of our eyes for a more open focus, giving us better peripheral vision, developing the ability to activate PSNS at critical points in time must be very useful indeed.

This has in fact been the foundation of Dr Rauch's groundbreaking research (as yet published only as a conference proceeding) carried out with athletes in Cape Town. Having identified a relationship between subtle, defensive postural adjustments under pressure and collapsing HRV (the 'choke' effect), he established a unique physical training protocol specifically designed to nullify the SNS overdrive in a physically stressful encounter (for example, sparring in boxing). The tool he used to do so was posturally correct movement, so it is no surprise that he worked with t'ai chi expert André Oelofse (who demonstrates some of the key sequences in *The Big Fat Fix*).

Although often perceived as a series of slow movements you might see crowds of older Asian folks enjoying in public spaces, t'ai chi is in fact a devastatingly effective ancient martial art. One of the purest martial arts, its lineage can be traced directly back to the battlefields of thousands of years ago.

When I had the opportunity to train with André (using the ten-session 'Calm in the Storm' syllabus he and Dr Rauch put together for the scientific study in Cape Town), to begin with, I found the movements clunky and awkward. On the seventh session, that all changed. As we were sparring, I noticed that my vision had widened, my movement was more fluid and it had become much easier for me to defend and avoid contact than before. It was as if everything was happening in slow motion around me. With my body loose and my mind fully alert, I was completely immersed in what sportspeople call 'the zone'.

The reason I was able to get into that zone was because my movement had become posturally correct – I had now learned to move from my spine. As a result of that, my pulse and breathing rates had reduced and my HRV had increased. My body's 'hard' defensive mode had been replaced with a vastly superior calmness.

By training with a series of posturally correct movement

sequences, my perception and management of the stressor facing me (André in his boxing gloves) had improved to the extent that the nervous energy so prevalent in our earlier sessions had disappeared. I now trusted my body, and felt safe.

Earlier, I was on the defensive 'back foot' and I did not feel 'safe', which increased my nervous energy. However, as proven by Dr Rauch's research, the posturally correct movement training took me to a place where I felt calm, safe and therefore free of nervous energy.

On top of that, my ability to make split-second decisions and respond to an attacking threat was greatly improved. I was operating from a place of much greater authority over my own movements and was in a better place to influence the outcome of the stress event in my favour (that is, to avoid being hit).

Based on my own experience, it comes as no surprise at all that t'ai chi has been proven to lengthen telomeres. So if, at any time, you feel edgy for no particular reason, try to neutralize that feeling with a natural movement sequence. The basic t'ai chi training movement (Day 8) in our Twenty-one-day Movement Protocol will help you do just that.

Remember, as André says in *The Big Fat Fix*, 'If you move (posturally) correctly from the spine, you breathe properly' – and, over time, the consequences of this are increased HRV and longer telomeres.

So, while we may not have access to the environment and *diaita* of Pioppi, we can still take steps (literally!) to optimize our response to our own day-to-day stressors.

By stepping away from your desk every forty-five minutes and moving around for a few moments, you can create an opportunity to focus on your breathing and posture simply by walking to the bathroom. Every step you take is an opportunity to think about making a fluid movement, breathing slowly, reducing your heart rate and increasing your HRV.

Think of those cues that were used with Aseem ('Let the shoulders relax, breathe slowly'; 'Think of a plumbline through the top of the head') and layer in Louise's walking tips ('Use the feet as pumps'; 'Really roll over the foot') to elevate your HRV instantly, then take it up a notch by blending in your basic t'ai chi movement every now and then throughout your day.

Stuck in traffic? Focus on your breathing and posture: 'Length through the back of the neck'; 'Soft in the jaw and throat'; 'Breathe in for five and out for five.' Waiting in a queue? Start with your feet and consciously work your way up through your body: 'Sway gently back and forward until you find a happy spot for your weight through your feet'; 'Relax the knees'; 'Tilt your pelvis marginally up and down until you find a happy place'; 'Breathe into the stomach, release any tension in the spine, shoulders and neck as you exhale'; 'Feel your arms heavy by your sides, fingertips heavy and relaxed.'

Once you learn to recognize and habitually manage your response to a stressor, it will help you on your journey to better health. In the same way that those seemingly innocuous, unrelated events can aggregate to establish a pattern of chronic stress, you can turn that around by nipping those situations in the bud in the first instance, then layering some simple HRV practice into your day (the US Navy Seals apparently teach their recruits to do this). Over time, these simple, powerful habits will not just help you keep those telomeres long and your HRV high, but your cognitive performance will also improve.

In summary:

- Stress can be a positive motivating force but, more often than not – for example, when you're sitting in traffic and running late – stress is a negative force

- Chronic stress is known to affect telomeres, an essential part of human cells that affect how our cells age

- The autonomic nervous system (ANS) is made up of two 'separate' systems: the ('fight or flight') sympathetic nervous system (SNS) and the ('rest and recovery') parasympathetic nervous system (PSNS). To manage stress effectively, we must learn to maintain the balance between the two systems

- Posturally correct movement and breathing sequences can help us to maintain that balance

13.

Intermittent Fasting

Fasting: 'to abstain from all or some kinds of food or drink, especially as a religious observance'

Intermittent fasting (IF): 'to regularly abstain from all or some kinds of food or drink except during a time-restricted eating window'

One of our keys objectives in visiting Pioppi was to identify elements of the traditional Mediterranean *diaita* that may have slipped through the cracks of time and the hands of science. When Antonio mentioned in passing that the men would have occasionally gone to work in the fields without food – effectively, in a fasted state – our ears pricked up immediately.

It is in this context that Aseem refers in *The Big Fat Fix* to the great work being done by Dr Jason Fung. Dr Fung has a clinic in Toronto, Canada, and is a leading global authority on the use of medically supervised fasting protocols for the management and reversal of type-2 diabetes. Should you wish to explore this topic in detail, he gives many excellent, in-depth presentations and interviews on YouTube, and I would encourage you to take a look.

For now, let's focus on the implications of mimicking the experience of food restriction in Pioppi by skipping meals occasionally and/or eating within a time-restricted window. The first point I would make is that both men and women would have experienced this kind of occasional fasting, because it was imposed by circumstance (lack of food), not through choice.

Pioppi was a very poor region in the post-war era, so the availability of food would have borne no resemblance whatsoever to the 24/7 food environment we now inhabit. Indeed, the 'food, energy and hunger' narrative of today – driven as much by supposedly robust health messages courtesy of those marketing breakfast cereals, energy drinks and various fast-food brands – leaves no room for not eating. Breakfast is the most important meal of the day, right? And it's downright dangerous not to eat five or six times a day, lest you get hungry and your energy levels crash. The end.

But then, they would say that, wouldn't they?

If you break down the word itself, 'breakfast' simply means to 'break' an overnight 'fast' after sleeping. There was never any golden rule suggesting that this must be done immediately upon waking, so what happens if you extend your perfectly natural overnight fast? Does it make any difference whether you do so by choice or whether circumstances have somehow dictated an absence of food?

How could the men of Pioppi have walked for miles, chopped wood and conducted a normal day's work without breakfast for 'fuel'?

The answer lies deep within our human DNA.

In his excellent book *The Complete Guide to Fasting*, Dr Fung points out that, despite the fact that we are constantly bombarded with messages to the contrary, 'There is no correlation whatsoever between constant eating and good health.'

The explosive growth in lifestyle diseases since the 1970s certainly supports this statement, but is there a clear relationship between good health and skipping meals or restricting eating windows, be it through conscious choice or otherwise?

The answer is a resounding yes. When you eat food, you are taking on board more energy than you need straight away, so your body must find a way to store the excess energy for later use.

As Aseem points out in Chapter 7, the conductor of this process is the hormone called insulin, which rises during meals in response to the stimulus provided by carbohydrates and protein (to a lesser extent) in your food. Fat has very little – if any – impact on insulin levels.

Insulin acts to allow you to access the fast, readily available energy from ingested carbohydrates. The carbohydrates you eat are turned into glucose almost immediately, raising your blood sugar levels; insulin then allows glucose to enter the various cells of the body, where it is (or at least should be) used for energy.

Ingested proteins are broken down into amino acids

and will not raise your blood sugar levels, but a variance in insulin response may occur. The fact that fats are not insulinogenic is one of the key reasons we recommend a higher-fat interpretation of the Mediterranean way of eating in the Pioppi Diet.

Any excess energy you have consumed can be stored by your body in one of two ways. Up to a point, glucose can be bundled up into glycogen (a multi-branched polysaccharide of glucose) for storage in the liver. When the liver's capacity to store glycogen is maxed out, your body must find another way to resolve the storage conundrum.

The process by which it does so is called de novo lipogenesis. This process turns the excess glucose into plain old fat, which can then be stored either in the liver itself or in fat deposits throughout the body. That there is essentially no limit to the amount of fat we can create via de novo lipogenesis perhaps goes some way towards explaining the explosion in global numbers of those classified as overweight and rates of obesity since the 1970s.

That excess has got to go somewhere, hasn't it?

Of course, it is logical and correct to assume that we can avoid the prospect of gaining fat simply by not eating, but that wouldn't be much fun either, would it? Interestingly, research shows that observing restricted eating windows – for example, you might consume your entire daily intake of food within a set eight-hour window each day – can be very effective in mimicking some of the benefits of fasting without actually fasting for prolonged periods of time.

In the month leading up to the Cape Town shoot for *The Big Fat Fix*, I followed this 'eight-hour eating window' protocol (popularized by the Swedish bodybuilder Martin Berkhan). By skipping breakfast and eating between noon and 8 p.m. each day, I was able to put on approximately one kilogram of muscle while marginally reducing my (already quite low) percentage of body fat.

The reason why this is so effective provides a glimpse of another key anti-ageing benefit the people of Pioppi enjoy, probably without even realizing it.

Within twenty-four hours of stopping eating, the body will respond with a 'health positive' hormonal storm. One of the most explicit benefits, which has attracted bodybuilders and athletes to this practice, is a spike in the production of human growth hormone (HGH).

This is interesting on a number of levels. Firstly, because growth hormone levels typically peak during puberty and then decrease gradually with age, the impact of very low levels of HGH (which include increased body fat, a marked reduction in lean muscle mass and decreased bone density) may only become apparent over several decades.

If it is possible to intermittently delay the decline in HRH by strategically timing your food intake now and then, why not? At forty-five, I am between the teeth of the ageing process, so any such tactics are certainly of interest to me. Fasting was something I had investigated as far back as 2010, when I was making *Cereal Killers*, but the science was then lacking for what at that time was essentially a preserve of the bodybuilding community.

As a side note, I have great respect for the bodybuilding community – they always seem to be ahead of the knowledge curve, and become so by literally putting their bodies on the line. One of the very best books I have read on the topic of fat adaptation is *The Anabolic Diet* by Dr Mauro Di Pasquale MD. A former world-champion powerlifter and competitive bodybuilder, Dr Pasquale wrote that book in the early 1990s explicitly for the bodybuilding community to promote a drug-free alternative to improve body composition. Twenty-five years later, it is clear that this publication was well ahead of its time.

To come back to HGH, another interesting point is the role it plays in signalling to the body to increase the availability of stored glucose (and results in higher blood sugar levels).

HGH is one member of a key group of counter-regulatory hormones (so called because they counter the effects of insulin), along with cortisol and adrenaline. This batch of powerful hormones typically 'pulse' (they are not secreted evenly through the day) loudest at 4 a.m., during your sleep cycle, in preparation for the day ahead.

All well and good, but what actual impact does this have on weight loss and ageing?

When we fast, our insulin levels drop and the body then responds to the signal to burn stored energy. First stop will be those glycogen stores in the liver, which are ample to tide us over for a day or so. After that, the next stop is stored body fat.

Of course, if we accept and follow the standard advice to keep eating and avoid those dreaded energy dips, we live permanently in the 'fed' state, which means our insulin levels remain high pretty much all the time.

Furthermore, because HGH increases glucose, it is naturally suppressed when we eat, meaning that the 'fed' state very effectively blocks out any prospect of those powerful, natural HGH spikes – and of course the myriad weight loss and anti-ageing benefits they offer – taking place. When Dr Fung points out that overeating can suppress total HGH secretion by up to 80 per cent, the potential impact on your health over several decades presents a compelling reason to at least consider fasting every now and then.

Dr Fung also points to one randomized controlled study from 1990 which suggests that the rewards may be quite exceptional. The study found that older people given HGH over a six-month period gained almost 4kg of lean muscle mass and lost an incredible 2.4kg of body fat. Viewed in this context, it is perhaps no surprise that externally administered HGH was one of the very first drugs to be abused by athletes seeking fast, illegal performance gains.

Great, except . . .

Those older folks who gained all that muscle and lost all that fat also increased their markers for myriad metabolic disorders, including heart disease and type-2 diabetes. While this seriously dilutes the appeal of a pharmaceutical, artificial HGH intervention, the good news is that interim studies have proved that fasting offers all the same benefits – and with none of the adverse side effects.

These benefits include:

- Improved body composition: an increase in lean muscle mass and a reduction in fat mass

- A less fatty liver

- Lower blood pressure

- Increased fat burning

- Increased insulin sensitivity

- Reduced inflammation

- Better cognitive function

Note: Many athletes today strategically deplete glycogen levels with the help of a very high-intensity session before training in a 'fasted' state in a bid for marginal training gains but, in practice, the easiest way for you to deplete glycogen is simply not to eat (i.e. to fast).

In fact, one recent study in Italy found 'an intermittent fasting program in which all calories are consumed in an 8-hour window each day, in conjunction with resistance training, could improve some health-related biomarkers, decrease fat mass, and maintain muscle mass in resistance-trained males'. Although this study did not do so, it would have been interesting to review HGH levels in the participants to see exactly what was happening in that context.[1]

If the recent trend for 'fasting diets' can be attributed to the genuine health benefits conferred by this perfectly normal state, the notion that you may eat with abandon when you are not fasting is an unhelpful perception. The Pioppi Diet, however, emphasizes the enjoyment of natural foods which are lower in carbohydrates and higher in healthy fats, and so your body will be much better equipped to let you fast comfortably for twenty-four hours, or to experiment with time-restricted eating for a few days – or for however long you wish to, if you are enjoying it.

By integrating intermittent fasting into your habitual lifestyle each week, you will be compounding the already exceptional benefits of the Pioppi Diet. The significant gains you can add to your cardiovascular, physical and mental health and longevity are real – and they are readily available to you.

Even if a stringent adherence to restricted eating windows is not necessarily practical for you, the good news is that you can simply choose to dip in and out of it – just as the people of Pioppi would have traditionally. For that reason, we recommend just one twenty-four-hour window of fasting each week. That might mean dinner on one evening, then consuming only fluids throughout the following day until dinner time twenty-four hours later.

When fasting, my own drink of choice is a coffee with coconut cream (it won't dilute the benefits coming your way), and that seems to carry me through really smoothly. If you have any concerns, rest assured: your body is designed to run perfectly well outside of that 'fed' state – counter to the messages we are constantly being given by the food industry and by many medical and nutrition 'experts'. It's not as difficult as you might think, and you may very well surprise yourself with just how good you feel. Make it a habit, and you've just added another free and easy – but very powerful – weapon to your anti-ageing arsenal.

In summary:

- Short periods of fasting were common in Pioppi (due to an occasional lack of food), but this was overlooked in the original research for the Mediterranean Diet

- We now know that intermittent fasting is a powerful health intervention

- When we fast, our insulin levels drop and the body then responds to the signal to burn stored energy

- The Pioppi Diet recommends fasting for twenty-four hours once a week

PART TWO
The Twenty-One-Day Plan

14.

The Guidelines

You've read the science. Now it's time to switch to the Twenty-One-Day Plan, and here are the reasons why.

1. It is full of nutritious, tasty food that makes you feel full and energized.

2. By shifting focus away from fear of fat towards insulin resistance and inflammation, it will help you:

   - lose excess body fat

   - reduce the risk of developing type-2 diabetes

   - manage or reverse impaired blood glucose conditions

   - reduce high medication loads, and prevent and treat heart disease

   - get you on the road to significantly reducing your risk of developing dementia and cancer

Enjoy . . .

- Three meals a day and eat until you feel full

- At least two to four tablespoons of extra virgin olive oil daily

- One small handful of tree nuts (walnuts/almonds/hazelnuts/macadamias) daily

- At least five to seven portions of fibrous vegetables and low-sugar fruits a day. We suggest one or two pieces of fruit and at least five vegetables a day (see Aseem and Donal's Top-Ten Foods). For potatoes opt for the sweet variety and if you're overweight or have type-2 diabetes try to limit consumption to no more than two portions a week!

- Vegetables with at least two meals daily, preferably three.

Avoid . . .

- All added sugars (it's everywhere, check those labels!), fruit juice, honey and syrups

- All packaged, refined carbohydrates, in particular anything flour based, including bread, pastries, cakes, biscuits, muesli bars, packaged noodles, pasta, couscous and rice

- Industrial seed oils typically used for cooking (i.e. no sunflower, canola, rice bran, corn or soya bean oil)

If you're really struggling with a desire for something sweet or you're missing your usual dessert with your evening meal, satisfy your craving with a piece of fruit. From week three, you can introduce a square of dark chocolate, like Aseem has with his morning coffee. We recommend chocolate with greater than 85 per cent cocoa solids, as it has the least amount of added sugar.

After week three, you will have had enough time experiencing life without sugar and refined carbohydrates. You may decide that you miss bread, pasta and rice, and you may not. If you do, we advise you to think of them as treats to have infrequently, in small amounts – and, most importantly, to listen to your body.

Red Meat

The World Cancer Research Fund recommends a maximum weekly limit of 500g of red meat. There are concerns that over-consumption of red meat could increase the risk of colon cancer. Although this still remains a controversial area, we advise you to stick within that limit: you don't want red meat to replace all the positive health benefits gained from the foods that form the base of the Pioppi Diet. Ideally, opt for meat from grass-fed animals. We would advise exercising some caution around processed red meats and focusing more on the whole-food, less processed varieties. Even with these limits, you can still enjoy a weekend fry-up with a couple of rashers of bacon or sausages, and some bolognese courgetti, a lamb curry or a juicy, nutritious eight-ounce steak during the week.

Fast

For one twenty-four-hour period each week you will not eat, i.e. you will fast. This is best done by eating as normal until the end of the day, and then not eating breakfast or lunch the next day. Consume fluids such as tea, coffee or sparkling water only during this time. We advise you to do this, to begin with, on day six to seven. Note: missing a meal does not mean that you should make up for it with your next meal by overeating.

Can I Follow the Pioppi Diet if I'm Vegetarian?

Absolutely YES! The key is to avoid refined carbohydrates and industrial seed oils and to ensure that you're taking in the daily amount of extra virgin olive oil and a small handful of nuts. Indulge in non-starchy vegetables and low-sugar fruit to your heart's content.

Alcohol

As a nation, we British are consuming way too much alcohol. Remember from Chapter 4 that alcohol in excess has a similar metabolic effect on the body as sugar. So stick within the current recommended limits of fourteen units a week, and drink like they do in the Mediterranean – no more than one glass of red wine with your evening meal. At this level, alcohol may even prove beneficial, in protecting your heart, and eventually help you to drop dead healthy and happy. As they say in Pioppi, 'One glass a day is the way to heaven.'

Move

- Do not sit for more than forty-five minutes at a time – take two-minute mini movement breaks

- Walk for at least thirty minutes five days a week, and make sure it's a brisk one. Mix up the pace for even greater benefits

- Spend as much time as possible outdoors in and around nature (for example, in parks or forests), and take the stairs wherever possible

- Increase your movement by parking further away from the entrance to the shopping centre/office, etc.

- Learn to move better – try the Twenty-One-Day Movement Protocol

Breathe

To reduce your stress levels, do a breathing exercise daily. Breathe in for five seconds, then out for five seconds, for two minutes four times a day. Be mindful and focus *only* on your breathing during this time.

Socialize

Make an effort to increase the time you spend with friends and family each week. Smile and laugh as much as you can.

Sleep

Aim for a minimum of seven hours each night. Reduce exposure to blue light (phones, computers, etc.) for at least two hours before bedtime.

15.

The Movement Protocol

(Developed with and written by Louise Knoop O'Neill of Prime Movement.)

Guiding factors:

- Listen to your bones – they fit together in very specific ways. If a joint feels like it is going to scream, back off to find its optimal zone for the movement sequence.

- Do not confuse muscular intensity for joint discomfort – muscles are made to move us. Listen to the cues and allow your arm and leg muscles to bear your weight.

- If your jaw and teeth are involved, the intensity of the movement sequence is above *your* normal.

- Each day of movement builds on the days before. If you are on Day 13 and the movement sequence for that day does not feel right for your joints, refer back to a previous day's sequence that targets the same joints.

Day 1
Chi (helicopter) arms

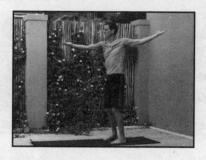

Feet parallel in supportive stance.

Knees soft.

Pelvis steady.

Arms stretched out to each side at shoulder height or just below, palms up.

Rotate the ribcage with the arms from side to side, looking for space to breathe wide, rolling your ribcage around your lungs, around your twisting spine.

Keep the gaze soft and the head balanced over the ribcage, over the pelvis, over the knees, and steady feet throughout.

Day 2
Four-point kneeling circles into walking-on-the-spot plank

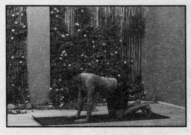 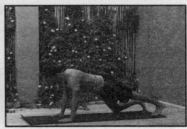

Set the hands wider than the shoulders, spreading all five fingers, index finger pointing forward and slightly out.

Knees underneath the hips or the belly. Distribute your weight in a way that makes your wrist, hip and knee joints comfortable.

For further support, tuck the toes under, pressing weight on to the balls of the feet.

Circle your stable torso in one direction a few times; reverse and circle in the opposite direction.

Look for good movement around the shoulder socket, the hip socket and the wrist joint.

From there, actively stand into one foot, preparing for plank by pushing into the support on the ball of that foot. Do the same with the other foot. Distribute your weight in a way that makes your wrists, shoulders and lower back comfortable.

Start walking on the spot, finding a push and pull between the opposing movements – one knee bending slightly while the other leg lengthens behind you. Push off your hands and arms and press into your feet to find the strength you need to support the entirety of your plank and to bear your own weight.

Keep the chest proud, crown of the head forward.

Stretch into alternate calf muscles throughout the sequence.

Day 3
Chi feet

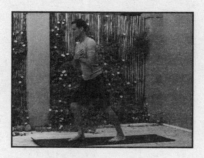

Place the feet parallel, hip width apart. Move your right leg forward about 30 centimetres. Each foot should be in its own track, in line with its own hip joint.

Transfer your weight on to the front leg with a soft knee, and back to the back leg with a bent knee.

As you move on to the front (right) foot, the back (left) leg will straighten, and vice versa.

Hip bones remain parallel and facing forward.

Head, ribcage and pelvis move as one unit between this weight-transference exercise.

Become aware of the full power of the feet by spreading the toes and really feeling the balls of the feet. Keep the heel grounded throughout.

Day 4
Squat

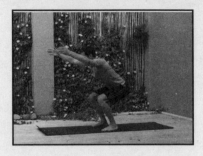

Place the feet parallel, slightly wider than hip width apart.

Sit down into your hips, knees and ankle joints and propel yourself out of that sit.

Reach the arms forward to counterbalance.

Keep energy out the crown of the head and the sitting bones.

Allow your gaze to shift down to the ground during the squat and back upright out of the squat, maintaining your head, ribcage and pelvis as one unit throughout the sequence.

Allow your joints to fold into the squat, and push out of it.

Track your knees directly over your toes.

Day 5
Plank to V

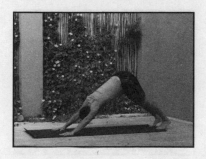

Collarbones wide, jaw released throughout.

From the four-point kneeling position, actively step each foot out into the plank.

Press the pelvis up above your feet by pushing into the arms and creating an inverted V with your body (or downward-facing dog).

Pull yourself forward into one long plank.

Again, find the push up into the V position and pull back into plank.

Push into the hands and the heels (as much as your joints allow).

Pull forward into a plank position that feels like it is flying.

Energy from the crown of the head in the plank to the tailbone in the V. Drop the head slightly in the V so that the back of the neck feels longer in the plank.

Day 6
Lunge

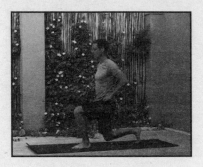

Start at the back of your space.

Place the feet parallel, hip width apart.

Step forward with one foot as you lunge and bend into both knees.

Push out of the lunge and back to parallel stance.

Alternate your lunges, making sure to step quite far forward for good alignment of the front knee over the ankles, rather than the foot.

Dip the back knee down to the ground (or close to it) to a point at which you can propel out of the movement with pure leg strength.

Keep the hip bones square. (A good tip is to keep the hands on the hips.)

Use the propulsion through the back foot to help you return to parallel stance.

The front leg is active on the step forward; the back leg provides the power to return to parallel stance.

Day 7
Spine roll

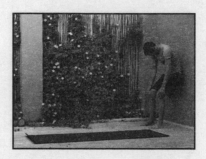

Keep the shoulders wide throughout.

Lean the torso against the wall with the feet about a foot away from the wall. (Make sure you are not on a slippery surface.)

The head need not touch the wall, but it should be easily balanced on the spine.

With strong feet and soft knees, start to roll the chin to the chest and peel the spine off the wall vertebra by vertebra, rib by rib.

To return, press into the heels to roll the pelvis back on to the wall, then press through your arches to restack your organs and spine on to the wall, and then on to the balls of the feet to balance the shoulders and head in the upright position.

Repeat a few times.

To come away from the wall, first bring the feet underneath you, then step away from the wall.

Day 8
Basic tai chi movement from *The Big Fat Fix*

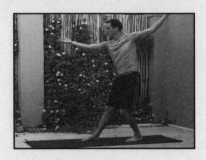

Keep the gaze soft, the hips forward and the breathing easy but expansive.

Start with the feet as with chi feet (Day 3): parallel, in their own tracks, one foot forward.

The front leg is bent and the back leg straight.

Start to swing the arms and rotate the ribcage, as in chi (helicopter) arms (Day 1), palms up.

Once you have a good feeling doing this rotation movement, do three swings with the weight on the front leg and three swings moving your weight to the back leg, and so on.

Change legs and repeat.

Day 9
Knee stretches

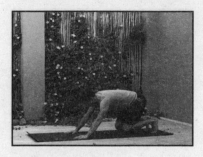

Back into four-point kneeling, with the hands just wider than the shoulders.

Keep the knees underneath the hips.

Tuck the toes under and keep the weight on the balls of the feet.

Press into the arms and feet and lift the knees just off the ground.

Push off the hands and sit your sitting bones back towards the heels.

Return to centre.

Push back and rebound forward a little. (Not a lot – this is a weight-bearing, deep squat.)

The accent is on the sit, not on the forward motion, keep it contained within the shape constructed by your arms and feet.

Keep active through the base of the big toes to keep the knees in parallel alignment.

The spine is in neutral – one long line from the crown of head to the sitting bones.

And *breathe*!

Day 10
Mountain climbers

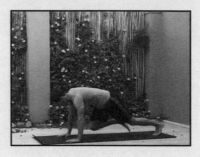

Actively step yourself out into a plank, hands wide underneath the shoulders.

From walking on the spot, pick up the pace to running on the spot by drawing one knee in at a time, with a swift and smooth interchange, while pressing into the elasticity of a calf stretch on the other leg.

Breathe evenly and jump through your joints.

Day 11
Basic crawl

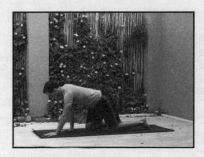

From four-point kneeling with the toes tucked under, begin to crawl forward a few 'steps', and then back.

Don't think about it too much to start with – allow the body's natural intelligence to remember the forward and reverse motions of crawling.

Once you have given that a go, aim to move the opposite arm and leg forward and then back at the same time.

It doesn't need to feel too linear, as if you are crawling along a tightrope. Allow integrated movements throughout the limbs and torso, maybe even then a consequent manoeuvre from side to side as you move forward and back.

Day 12
Lunge walks forward and back

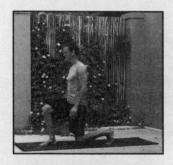

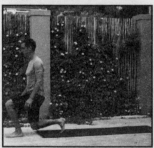

Place the feet parallel, hip width apart.

Keep the hips square throughout.

As with the lunge (Day 6) take a large step forward to lunge, with both knees bent.

Push off the back foot to immediately step forward into another lunge, with both knees bent.

Repeat a few times: forward lunge right leg, then forward lunge left leg; then left leg to back lunge, then right leg to back lunge.

Keep the hands either on the hips or swing both arms forward to counterbalance each lunge.

Day 13
Four-point kneeling, oiling the ankles

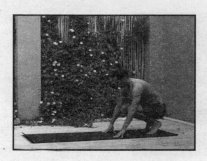

From four-point kneeling, walk the hands closer to the knees as you push your weight back into a very deep, parallel and primitive squat.

Roll forward and back on the feet, mobilizing deeply into the hip, knee and ankle joints.

Maintain parallel knees in alignment with the hips and ankles. Make sure not to knock the knees.

Place the hands on a yoga brick, or something similar, if you find the lower back under strain to touch the ground.

Day 14
Dog to cat spine

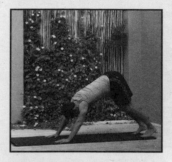

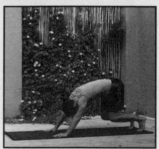

From four-point kneeling, press the pelvis up into an inverted V, but keep the knees remain soft so that you can stretch the spine into a gentle arch.

Bend the knees and round the spine into an angry-cat spine.

Press back into the V, looking more for a chest stretch than a hamstring stretch.

Round your ribs up to the sky for a round spine stretch.

With care to keep the knees slightly bent throughout, try to move your spine as much as possible through the two very different movements of extension (arching) and flexing (rounding).

Day 15
Dynamic crawling

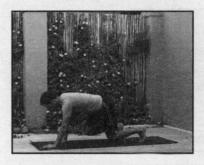

From four-point kneeling, tuck the toes under, and using the balls of your feet lift your knees just off the ground.

Move forwards, using the opposite arm to the leg a few times, then reverse the crawl, moving backwards, using the opposite arm to the leg a few times.

As you get the hang of it, you will feel certain joint bounces happening as you find your propulsion, as in the knee stretches (Day 9).

Allow your body to move forwards and backwards with natural intent.

Day 16
Tabata timer

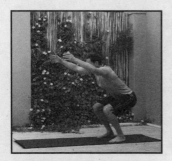

Four minutes of high-intensity effort (twenty seconds of maximal effort – followed by ten seconds' rest, repeated eight times) using the Tabata Timer app, do:

Squats, knee stretches or plank to knee stretches.

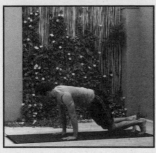

Day 17
Reverse crawl

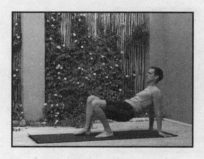

Start in a reverse four-point kneeling position, then

sit with the feet in front of you, knees bent.

Hold the arms straight out behind you.

Lift the tailbone just off the ground and begin to 'walk' forwards and backwards, using the opposite arm to the leg.

Allow a bit of sway to find your rhythm.

(Those with shoulder problems, please take care. It is better to stay in the static position and build weight-bearing strength in this open position prior to crawling.)

Day 18
Chi feet and arms – lunging and walking

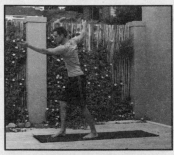

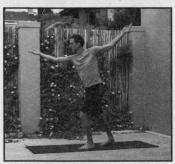

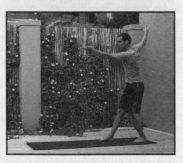

To 'walk' backwards:

Parallel feet, right foot forward in chi lunge.

Begin swinging chi (helicopter) arms in forward lunge of right leg.

Keep swinging arms, transfer weight to back left foot.

Still swinging arms step back with right leg.

Keep swinging arms, transfer weight to back right foot.

Still swinging arms, step back with left leg.

(each foot movement, be it a step or a weight transfer has 3 arm swings)

To 'walk' forward:

Begin swinging chi (helicopter) arms in forward lunge of right leg.

Keep swinging arms, keep weight on right leg, left foot forward.

Keep swinging arms, transfer weight to front left foot.

Still swinging arms, keep weight on left leg, step forward with right leg.

Keep swinging arms, transfer weight to front right foot.

(each foot movement, be it a step or a weight transfer, has 3 arm swings).

Day 19
Dynamic squats

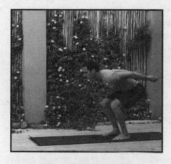

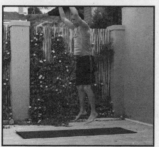

Begin in a small squat, with the feet parallel, a little wider than hip width apart.

Stand upright on to the balls of the feet, swinging the arms up as you rise on to the toes.

As you rise, press through the ball of the foot to activate calf pump, sending blood back up to your heart.

Swing the arms down and wide as you sit back into the squat.

This should naturally progress into a small jump: use the balls of the feet as propulsion and land on the toes, balls of the feet and heel as a natural stabilizer.

Jump with the legs, not with the torso.

Day 20
Warrior squat to lunge to warrior

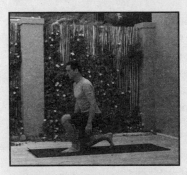

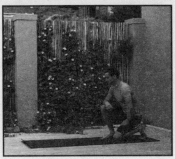

This is a progression of your lunges (Day 6), ankle oiling (Day 13) and squats (Day 4).

Start by lunging forward on your left leg, dipping the right knee towards the ground.

Step back out of the lunge with the left leg to sit right down into a warrior squat: the pelvis sits on the left heel (toes tucked under with the weight on the ball of the left foot); the right leg is bent in front of the body, the right foot flat on the ground.

Repeat a few times: left leg lunge forward and the left leg step back and sit into a warrior squat.

Change legs to start with right leg lunge forward, step the right leg back and sit back into warrior squat.

Day 21
Evolution crawl

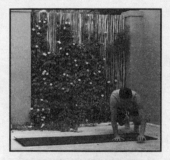

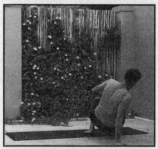

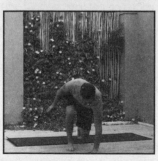

Start in the four-point kneeling position.

Lift the knees, tuck the toes under to bear the weight on the balls of the feet.

Crawl forward two steps, using opposite arm and leg.

Crawl, then tumble sideways by opening the front body to the sky, transferring the weight between the limbs as you go to transition to an upright walk forward for a few steps.

Repeat, starting with the opposite arm and leg.

Crawl with the right hand and the left leg.

Crawl with the left hand and the right leg.

Crawl, then tumble on to the right hand and swing the left leg over.

Land on the left hand and step forward with the right leg, to walk naturally.

Crawl with the left hand and the right leg.

Crawl with the right hand and the left leg.

Crawl, then tumble on to the left hand and swing the right leg over.

Land on the right hand and step forward with the left leg, to walk naturally.

Go for it! Crawl, crawl, tumble, tumble, walk, walk . . . repeat.

16.

Aseem and Donal's Top-ten Foods

1. Extra virgin olive oil

Prescription: 2 to 4 tablespoons daily

There are many robust, science-based reasons why we recommend two to four tablespoons of extra virgin olive oil. It is one of the healthiest foods for your heart and general health, and the list of benefits is endless. It reduces inflammation and prevents high blood pressure, especially when combined with vegetables. It improves the function of the endothelium (the lining of the blood vessels), which is where the development of heart disease begins, prevents LDL cholesterol particles from oxidizing (becoming damaging) and improves the post-prandial, or 'after eating' blood glucose response to food (preventing blood sugar spikes). Olive oil also contains very little in the way of omega-6 fatty acids, a group of fatty acids that are particularly rife in modern diets and which can increase inflammation.

In Pioppi, we learned that the locals who consumed at least four tablespoons of extra virgin olive oil a day would, traditionally, have grown and pressed their own olives locally to produce this elixir of good health – a stark contrast to the mass-produced, industrially processed seed and vegetable oils which need to be bleached, deodorized and chemically processed for an end product to be extracted. The first press was considered to be the highest quality – extra virgin – with the second press typically used as a cooking oil in the home. Today, the process has been expedited, but don't be fooled by marketing terms such as 'cold pressed'; instead, do your homework and understand which brands are 100 per cent extra virgin olive oil. Unfortunately, mislabelling remains prevalent.

It has been suggested that olive oil is not stable for cooking, but the science tells us otherwise. However, one study, in which it was heated to 180°C (or 356°F) for thirty-six hours, demonstrated significant stability in heat. This is because it contains mostly monounsaturated (double bonded) fatty acids. No surprise, then, to see Chef Antonio pouring it generously into his pan in the kitchen of Suscettibile! Top tip: if you do want to stabilize it further, just add a knob of butter.

By making extra virgin olive oil the basis of your natural fat intake, you are laying an excellent foundation for improved health – just be sure to invest in a quality brand. It not only tastes great, but it is incredibly calorie dense and, all things considered, remarkably cost effective when you consider the bang for your buck – and your health.

2. Nuts

Prescription: a handful daily

Nuts are a wholesome and highly nutritious wholefood, packed with monounsaturated fats and powerful health benefits. Many studies have replicated the finding that nuts can significantly improve lipid profiles and reduce the total cholesterol to HDL ratio. But, beyond affecting cholesterol, the greatest benefits of nuts are most likely their anti-inflammatory qualities, which are also well documented in the literature. The participants in the PREDIMED study enjoyed a 35 per cent decrease in C Reactive Protein (CRP), which is a marker of inflammation in the body. Perhaps even more impressively, that same study also reported a 90 per cent decrease in interleukin 6 (IL-6), another key marker of inflammation. And that's not all. People with metabolic syndrome or type 2 diabetes have experienced improvements in blood sugar control when prescribed nuts, and the impact of your daily handful on arterial function is possibly even superior to that of extra virgin olive oil. Small wonder, then, that 90,000 deaths each year could be prevented in the US alone with this simple prescription!

Let's not forget the abundance of very high-quality fibre – which you absolutely won't find in 'wholegrain' breakfast cereals! – in nuts, either. In addition to the aforementioned metabolic benefits, that fibre gets turned into short-chain fatty acids (SCFAs) in the gut, which then nourishes that oh-so-important bacteria in there. Almonds were prevalent in Pioppi: rest assured that any unprocessed, raw nuts are a great option. Just don't go crazy on volume and think of that small handful as both a limit and a guide. The nuts we recommend in particular are tree nuts. In PREDIMED, the participants were advised to consume, in total, 30g a day: of walnuts (15g), almonds (7.5g) and hazelnuts (7.5g).

3. Fibrous vegetables

Broccoli

Arguably packing the greatest nutritional punch, this cruciferous green has the highest concentration of immune-boosting vitamin C than any vegetable. It's also a great source of folate, vitamin K and calcium and is high in soluble fibre. Like other non-starchy vegetables, it's consumption is associated with a reduced risk of cancers of the mouth, throat and stomach.

In a double-blind randomized controlled test of a small group of patients with type-2 diabetes, consumption of 10g a day of broccoli-sprout powder led to significant reductions in triglycerides, oxidized LDL cholesterol and increased HDL cholesterol within just four weeks.

Cauliflower

In addition to being a great substitute for high-glycaemic white rice when blended, cauliflower, the cruciferous twin of broccoli, is also high in vitamin C and folate and is a great source of magnesium, phosphorus, thiamin, vitamin B6 and soluble fibre.

Courgettes

Our substitute for spaghetti, this popular staple vegetable of Pioppi is abundant in soluble fibre (in the peel) and is also an excellent source of potassium, which counteracts the effects of a high sodium intake to help lower blood pressure.

Aubergines

Another high-fibre vegetable, the aubergine is full of anti-oxidants, in particular nasunin, which gives the skin its purple appearance. Nasunin has been found to protect brain cell membranes.

Onions

Forming the base of many dishes across the Mediterranean regions and Asia, onions are known for being particularly high in flavonoids. Flavonoids are phytonutrients (plant chemicals) with powerful antioxidant and anti-inflammatory benefits. Flavonoids can also be considered as cardioprotective, due to their interaction with the endothelium. They are taken up by endothelial cells and cause a rise in nitric oxide expression. This helps the endothelium to become more resilient to damage, and also causes the smooth muscle of the vessel walls to relax, helping to reduce blood pressure.

Sweet potatoes

A staple of the centenarians of the Japanese island of Okinawa, sweet potato has more fibre and a lower glycaemic index than regular white potato. Furthermore, the flesh is packed with carotenoids, the substances responsible for its bright orange colour. These are a group of fat-soluble antioxidants, which means they naturally migrate to the fatty tissues of the body. This is what makes carotenoids so good for the skin. They can accumulate in the subcutaneous layer of the skin and offer localized antioxidant protection to structures like collagen and elastin, which help give the skin its structural integrity.

However, if you suffer from type-2 diabetes, we recommend that you don't exceed more than two portions a week during the Twenty-one-day Plan.

4. Fruits

Tomatoes

Perhaps the most popular staple of Italian and Indian cuisine, the health benefits tomatoes offer are most likely due to their lycopene content. Lycopene is an antioxidant that has been linked to reduced incidence of heart disease and cancer.

Avocados

One of the most nutrient-dense low-sugar fruits, avocados, which are high in monounsaturated fats, contain almost twenty vitamins and minerals, as well as having one of the highest fibre contents of any fruit, at 7g per 100g.

Apples

Apples are another fruit very rich in antioxidants, flavonoids and dietary fibre, and numerous studies have demonstrated that regular consumption is associated with a reduction in the risk of dementia. One study, carried out by researchers at the University of Oxford, suggested that an apple a day was as effective as statin drugs in preventing heart attack or stroke in those aged over fifty.

Berries

Blueberries, blackberries and raspberries are all rich sources of flavonoids. As outlined earlier, these antioxidant compounds are very beneficial for cardiovascular health, as they can help to protect the inner lining of vessels from inflammatory damage, and relax vessel walls to reduce pressure within the vessel.

5. Herbs and spices

Garlic

This was a secret favourite of Ancel Keys: we learned in Pioppi that he would consume one raw clove, taken like a pill, daily. It certainly didn't appear to do him any harm, as he lived to the age of 100. Garlic is enriched with vitamin B6 (pyridoxine) and is a great source of vitamin C, selenium, manganese, phosphorus, iron and copper. Although it is known to reduce total and LDL cholesterol without affecting HDL cholesterol, its benefit most likely comes from its abundance of the antioxidant compounds alliin, allyl cysteine, allyl disulphide and allicin.

Ginger

A flavoursome flowering plant popularly used in Asian cuisine, ginger provides a high concentration of the essential nutrient and mineral manganese, in addition to being an excellent source of iron, magnesium and zinc. It's also high in niacin and vitamin B6. Manganese has an important role in maintaining a healthy bone structure and also acts to assist in human metabolism.

Turmeric

This spice is a staple of Indian cuisine and has been very widely studied globally. The orange/yellow colour pigments in turmeric (curcuminoids) have been shown to offer anti-inflammatory activity. They interact with an enzyme called cyclo-oxygenase, which is involved in converting the fatty acid arachidonic acid into the pro-inflammatory series-2 prostaglandin (prostaglandins are a group of compounds that act like hormones.)

Basil

Basil is packed with a wide array of antioxidants. It has been used in western herbal medicine for centuries as a remedy for infections of the intestinal tract, and it is believed its fragrant flavour derives from the essential oils present in it.

Cinnamon

Cinnamon is another spice with a vast and complex anti-oxidant profile. There is a traditional use of cinnamon as a circulatory stimulant, and to ease bloating.

6. Fatty fish

Prescription: lots! Minimum 3 times a week

Fish is a bit like sleep. Everyone knows it's a great option, but most of us don't get enough. If all fish offers a high-quality protein option – with the added bonus of iodine, and myriad vitamins and minerals in there as well – fatty fish are top of the pile when it comes down to heart health.

Oily fish are the most superior and preferred source of omega-3 fatty acids. This is because they exist in the forms of EPA and DHA. Omega-3 is not one single nutrient but a family of fatty acids. The ones that feed into metabolic pathways and benefit our health are the long-chain EPA and DHA. We often hear how seeds like flax and chia are 'great sources of omega-3' – well, this is only a partial truth.

Yes, they are packed with omega-3 in the form of ALA; however, before this form of omega-3 is able to have any influence on our health, it needs to be converted by enzymes called desaturases and elongases into the longer-chain EPA and DHA. This is great in theory – until we realize that humans are very, very poor at performing this conversion: around a 6 per cent conversion rate of dietary ALA into EPA, and about a 0.5 per cent conversion into DHA. Not a good picture! This rate of conversion will never get you anywhere near a replete level. The only time this conversion changes is in pregnant women, where it ramps up to about 25 per cent. Animals such as fish that swim in upper layers of the water, and grazing cattle, can do this conversion of ALA into EPA and DHA much more efficiently, and then store these fatty acids in their tissue. So, by eating these foods, we can bypass this inadequate enzymatic pathway and just feed these metabolically active forms of omega-3 straight into where they need to go.

While the research has focused closely on the powerful omega-3 fatty acids in these fish (including salmon, mackerel, sardines, anchovies), it's interesting to see that supplementing with these oils alone is now falling out of favour. That tells us there must be something else in the fish itself (which we have yet to identify) that is explicitly beneficial.

This knits in very well with the 'food as medicine' philosophy of the Pioppi Diet, and the recipes given reflect our strong preference for fish as a protein option.

If the science is robustly supportive of the health benefits of high-quality fatty fish, then so too are the people of

Pioppi. The fishing boats leaving the village every day return with an outstanding bounty and we enjoyed an excellent and diverse array of seafood while we were there, including sardines, tuna and even octopus. This is one wonderful custom that has not changed at all since the era of Ancel Keys. The boats fish in pristine waters for that which the locality requires – and no more.

7. Dark chocolate (85 per cent cocoa solids, or more) and/or raw cacao powder

Prescription: 30g a day, or 1 tablespoon of raw cacao/ cocoa

Note: premium cocoa powder is 22–24 per cent fat, twice the amount of regular cocoa powder – so do check the label.

Endothelial function, improvements in blood pressure and insulin sensitivity and an abundance of polyphenols all merit consideration when discussing the proven health attributes of dark chocolate and/or cacao consumption.

Studies have, in fact, demonstrated a range of significant outcomes, from lowered blood pressure and improved insulin sensitivity (for subjects eating dark chocolate for fifteen days) to protection against oxidization of LDL cholesterol particles and increased HDL (for subjects eating cocoa powder), which points to some very powerful and easily accessible gains – just by eating chocolate! By extension, it is perhaps not surprising to see that chocolate consumption has also been inversely associated with the progression of atherosclerotic plaques in a study of 2,200 people.

They may not have consumed chocolate or cacao in Pioppi, but remember that the Pioppi Diet marries and merges the latest science with the wisdom of this region to create an enjoyable, sustainable and effective road to better health. In that regard, a little chocolate goes a long way. Just make sure that the label says 85 per cent cocoa solids or greater – and don't be afraid of the dark![1]

8. Coconut

Prescription: cook freely with coconut oil; try 1 teaspoon in your coffee (optional!)

Tip: as with olive oil, extra virgin coconut oil is a superior product option.

Once we set aside our misplaced fear of saturated fat, coconut can take its rightful place as a healthy, high-fat, wholefood option. In fact, populations which have traditionally consumed coconut – like the Tokelauans, who ate more than 50 per cent of their calorie intake in the form of coconut – display robust health and a much lower incidence of heart disease than any modern western society.

Coconut oil is 90 per cent saturated fat, but it is its fatty-acid structure which we are particularly interested in for health purposes. These fatty acids are called 'medium-chain triglycerides' (MCTs) and can go directly from the digestive tract to the liver, where they can be turned into an almost immediate source of energy for the body. As a quick point of reference, note that extra virgin olive oil consists predominantly of long-chain fatty acids (LCFAs), which do not offer this 'fast energy' option as the body must work a bit harder to break them down.

Aseem also likes the fact that coconut oil improves blood lipids by preferentially raising HDL cholesterol levels. With the added bonus of stability at very high cooking temperatures, you will often find him cooking his eggs in coconut oil or dropping a tablespoon into his morning coffee. Me? I prefer coconut cream!

9. Eggs

Prescription: minimum 10 a week

If eggs had a food label, it would be a long one. In addition to all nine essential amino acids – that's leucine, histidine, isoleucine, lysine, methionine, phenylalanine, threonine, tryptophan and valine accounted for – they contain vitamins A, D, E K, B2, B5, B6, B12, and folate, calcium, zinc, choline . . . and that list just keeps going. They really are a complete protein source, with a unique battery of vitamins, nutrients and health benefits.

Unfortunately, for many decades, eggs have been wrongly demonized. They were the perfect fall guy for the conventional cholesterol narrative which Aseem deconstructed earlier, which suggested that the cholesterol in eggs was in fact dangerous for heart health. Fortunately, we now understand that there is no correlation between egg consumption and heart disease, and any impact on lipid profiles may be compellingly positive. In that context, eggs have been shown to improve the structure of LDL subparticles, which reduces one's risk of developing cardiovascular disease.

The research now indicates that enjoying up to three eggs a day is not just perfectly safe but also a great way to source very high-quality protein in a tasty, power-packed package. If you don't have chickens in the yard, do look for higher-quality eggs – pasture-raised or organic – to maximize the bang for your buck. The superior omega-3 fatty-acid profile of eggs from these higher-quality sources (versus conventional battery-raised hens) is significant, so it's worth going the extra mile to find them.

10. Full fat and fermented dairy

Prescription: enjoy full-fat Greek yogurt, cheese and kefir, and cook with grass-fed butter

If dairy can be a controversial food group, then full-fat dairy has been the most controversial cohort of the lot. That being the case, it's important to clarify exactly what we are – and are not – recommending here.

All dairy is certainly not created equal. As infants, we produce a digestive enzyme called lactase to help break down lactose (the main carbohydrate in dairy) from our mother's milk. As we get older, many of us lose that ability, and this can lead to issues of lactose intolerance. That's common in African, Asian and South American populations, but much less so in Europe, North America and Australia.

Despite that, fermented dairy products (including yogurt, cheese and kefir) and butter are in fact well tolerated across the board and have a very high-quality nutrient composition that is quite different from milk, for example. That nutrient composition – and especially the fatty-acid composition – also depends very much on what the animals ate and the conditions in which they were raised.

Products derived from animals raised on grasslands have vastly superior omega-3 fatty-acid and vitamin K2 profiles than feedlot animals, and the same goes for the essential fatty acid conjugated linoleic acid (CLA) content – which you won't find in low-fat dairy products.

Studies of dairy consumption in countries where animals are predominantly grass-fed have repeatedly shown the health benefits of full-fat dairy consumption, and it is in this context that we recommend foods such as full-fat Greek yogurt, kefir and butter produced by grass-fed cattle. A recent Harvard study found that participants who consumed the most full-fat dairy products had less visceral fat, superior lipid results, lower levels of inflammation, better insulin sensitivity and a compelling 62 per cent lower risk of developing type-2 diabetes.

Although not prevalent in Pioppi, the Greek cohort in Ancel Keys's original studies enjoyed full-fat fermented dairy products and impeccable health markers as well – so there is no reason we shouldn't be doing likewise!

17.

A Week in the Life of the Pioppi Diet

While many diets can be restrictive and expensive, the Pioppi Diet is designed to fit your lifestyle – and your budget – wherever you are.

For example, if we consider not just the cost per calorie but also the quality of the product itself, then olive oil is one of the most cost-effective foods available to us. With a litre of good-quality oil available for less than £4 in the UK, those four tablespoons we recommend – amounting to almost 500 calories a day – cost less than twenty pence!

Once you make it the foundation of your food pyramid, the options with olive oil are extensive. It is not just an excellent medicinal food, it is also a tremendous option for cooking and dressing vegetables and salads, or drizzling on fish.

If extra virgin olive oil is a core foundation of the Pioppi Diet, then movement, sleep and stress reduction are also vitally important. And they're free!

In that context, Aseem and I thought we might share with you a glimpse of how we each observe the Pioppi Diet in our daily lives. After all, life for a cardiologist in

London is very different from that of a film-maker in Cape Town, but we each find ways to practise and enjoy the benefits of the lifestyle principles we share.

So, what exactly does a day in each of our lives look like? But before we get into the specifics, here's a bit of background.

Aseem – London

My love of good home-cooked food started in my early teens. Both my mum and my dad would cook almost every day, with perhaps once-a-week indulgences at the weekend at restaurants or of fast food. For religious reasons, my mum has been vegetarian most of her life, so we'd really only have meat at home during occasions when we'd have guests in the house, and it was usually in the form of my dad's famous chicken curry, which was passed down to him from his mother.

But I'm very lucky (and biased) because, when it comes to Indian vegetarian food, it can't be beaten either for taste or for variety of dishes. I could never get fed up with eating my dad's home-cooked dal or a vegetable curry. I later experimented with cooking what turned into my own vegetable curry, a dish originally based on Bombay's famous Pao Bhaji, a potato-based vegetable dish usually consumed with fried bread. However, since I completely cut out bread from my diet I've converted the bread element into a mix of sweet potato and various greens and I now eat it with cauliflower rice or just plain full-fat yogurt.

I've always enjoyed trying new recipes and have picked up so many different ones from my relatives and friends – even from the mum of my first girlfriend, who taught me how to make the most amazing pizza (now low-carb) sauce.

After my first year in halls of residence in university, I moved into a flat, and that's when I found myself cooking from scratch almost every evening after medical school lectures had finished. I find the process of cooking deeply relaxing, and cooking for others, be they friends or family, is even more fun.

Once I qualified as a doctor, in 2001, despite working late on calls in hospital, I'd never fail to cook my own food and, as I became more skilled over the years, I found I was able to cook various dishes in less than thirty minutes. Even when I was working nights and doing twelve-hour shifts seven days in a row, I'd fuel myself with some home-cooked food before driving off to the hospital. As I was only managing four hours' sleep at best during the day, and I was having to manage very sick patients in the middle of the night, I knew that keeping healthy was not only important for my own health but would affect my performance in the operating theatre. I owed that to my patients.

I also believe it's important to set the right example to patients. Sadly, the current obesity crisis also afflicts NHS staff, 50 per cent of whom are overweight or obese. I practise what I preach and consume my most important nutrients with a mix of Indian and Mediterranean cuisine.

Here's a typical food week for me.

	Monday	Tuesday	Wednesday
Breakfast	Single espresso mixed with 1 tablespoon of extra virgin coconut oil, 1 teaspoon of turmeric, 1 teaspoon of organic raw cacao powder and 1 teaspoon of ground cinnamon; 1 square of dark chocolate (85 per cent cocoa solids), a small handful of nuts and an apple	Single espresso mixed with 1 tablespoon of extra virgin coconut oil, 1 teaspoon of turmeric, 1 teaspoon of organic raw cacao powder and 1 teaspoon of ground cinnamon; 1 square of dark chocolate (85 per cent cocoa solids), a small handful of nuts and an orange	Single espresso mixed with 1 tablespoon of extra virgin coconut oil, 1 teaspoon of turmeric, 1 teaspoon of organic raw cacao powder and 1 teaspoon of ground cinnamon; 1 square of dark chocolate (85 per cent cocoa solids), a small handful of nuts and an orange
Brunch	1 fillet of smoked mackerel marinated in 2 tablespoons extra virgin olive oil; 2 hard-boiled eggs and a side of pickled cabbage	3-egg omelette cooked in extra virgin coconut oil with onions and tomatoes	2 fried eggs with avocado, spinach and a side of pickled cabbage
Dinner	Red kidney bean curry served with cauliflower rice, full-fat yogurt and Punjabi salad	Salmon curry served with Indian mixed vegetables (green beans, broccoli and cauliflower), full-fat yogurt and Punjabi salad	Tuna courgetti

Thursday	Friday	Saturday	Sunday
Fast until dinner; morning coffee before thirty-minute morning walk	Single espresso mixed with 1 tablespoon of extra virgin coconut oil, 1 teaspoon of turmeric, 1 teaspoon of organic raw cacao powder and 1 teaspoon of ground cinnamon; 1 square of dark chocolate (85 per cent cocoa solids), a small handful of nuts and an apple	Single espresso mixed with 1 tablespoon of extra virgin coconut oil, 1 teaspoon of turmeric, 1 teaspoon of organic raw cacao powder and 1 teaspoon of ground cinnamon; 1 square of dark chocolate (85 per cent cocoa solids), a small handful of nuts and a pear	Single espresso mixed with 1 tablespoon of extra virgin coconut oil, 1 teaspoon of turmeric, 1 teaspoon organic raw cacao powder and 1 teaspoon of ground cinnamon; 1 square of dark chocolate (85 per cent cocoa solids), a small handful of nuts and an apple
	Tuna Niçoise salad and tomato soup	Fry-up – 3 fried eggs, 2 rashers of bacon, avocado, mushrooms, spinach	3-egg omelette with avocado, mushrooms and a couple of sausages
Vegetable curry with full-fat yogurt and Punjabi salad	Karahi lamb with cauliflower and broccoli rice, full-fat yogurt and Punjabi salad	Low-carb pizza with pepperoni, onions, chillies and anchovies	Mediterranean mixed grill of fish with vegetables

Donal – Cape Town, South Africa

First thing every morning, I drink a glass of water with a tablespoon of apple cider vinegar in it; this is something I do before most meals and throughout the day. I do so because I enjoy it and because the blood glucose control benefits are well documented. My first coffee is strong (I use an old-fashioned Italian stove-top espresso maker), and I usually have it with coconut cream. My hunger is low in the morning so I tend to not eat breakfast during the week. By noon, I will typically have had three coffees, read the paper and spent a few hours in my creative zone, mapping out anything from a movie to a product design.

I will typically do some light movement every morning – a walk, body-weight exercises or whatever feels right. There is no prescription per se. I never do any HIIT, resistance training or sprints in the morning. Even when I was a competitive athlete, my early-morning performance was always poor, so I prefer to loosen up and park any harder work until later in the day. Until my body says yes, I say no – circadian rhythms are there to be obeyed!

My breakfast or brunch is typically egg-based. I find that three pastured hen eggs (fortunately, they are readily available here) is a perfect base for this meal. I have it with a choice between avocados, anchovies, bacon, tomato and – always – extra virgin olive oil. Anything cooked is done so with coconut oil, butter or extra virgin olive oil. A cup of Earl Grey tea and some dark chocolate – my favourite is a local 95 per cent cacao brand here – with a handful of nuts top that off.

An afternoon snack could be anything from canned oysters to pecans fried lightly in butter and coconut oil with Greek yogurt, coconut cream, berries and a sprinkle of cinnamon. If I am planning to do some sprints or an intense HIIT session that day, I might opt for a pre-training pancake made with an egg, a banana (preferably not too ripe) and a cinnamon and cacao mix. It's great served with those berries, Greek yogurt and/or coconut cream and gives me enough glycogen for a short but very intense workout. I have also used caffeine as a performance booster for myself and for the athletes I have been coaching now for twenty years. If you tolerate it well (there are genetic mechanisms at play in caffeine consumption, so not everyone does), it's effective.

Eating within an eight- to nine-hour window on weekdays really works for me, and I'm confident that's enough to confer the benefits of intermittent fasting we discussed earlier. One other little thing we enjoy is the home-made chicken-bone broth (made from the carcass of our weekly roast chicken dinner) we always have in our fridge – it's great with a shot of extra virgin olive oil, salt and black pepper. I will sometimes throw in canned mackerel or sardines with some coriander and spices to make a super-simple, tasty and nutritious fish soup.

The afternoon is probably my most constructive time of the day. I sit, then stand, then move around a lot – a 20kg kettlebell is always close by, for a random set of twenty kettlebell swings – while a pair of cats also do their best to distract me as much as possible from my keyboard. Who knew pets were such great little stress busters? Not me, until I married into them!

If I have not been outside, I will strive to do so before 4 p.m., to grab some vitamin D. Like many in the UK, I have tested low, but with the abundance of sunshine in South Africa, I prefer to get my daily dose outside rather than by taking a supplement.

A standard dinner for me is a huge raw salad: broccoli, seeds, spinach leaves, tomato, onion, with feta or Parmesan and some high-quality protein – hake fillets pan-cooked in olive oil or lamb loin chops are favourites – and a few sweet-potato chips oven-baked in coconut oil. The secret sauce is my wife's amazing, homemade 'yayonaise' – a blend of extra virgin olive oil, raw egg, feta, raw garlic, chilli and spices. After that, it's a cup of tea and a few more squares of that 95 per cent cocoa-solid chocolate or my home-made cacaonut bombs (raw cacao, coconut oil, cinnamon, cream and nuts heated then blended and frozen into bite-size pieces).

During the filming of *Cereal Killers* back in 2012, I consumed 50g of dark chocolate a day as part of that specific plan, and I have pretty much continued down the cacao track ever since. Just remember that 'chocolate' is a very loose term indeed, and the variance in sugar and cocoa content is enormous. Comparing that 95 per cent cocoa option with regular milk chocolate is like comparing a wild salmon to a McDonald's Filet-O-Fish burger. One is a quality food; the other is low-grade junk!

Late evening is the only time I spend – briefly – in a

completely sedentary state. We don't own a conventional sofa (they are poorly designed for bodies that like to move around) but crash out on our huge chaise longue to watch an episode of something completely ridiculous to tune out. My wife frequently tells me my thoughts are too loud, so it's always good to switch off for a bit

As darkness descends, my MacBook has the Flux app active so the screen brightness will respond to the time of day and dim accordingly to reduce my exposure to blue light. If I am on there for any reason, it's a really neat and effective little option – and free to download.

Before bedtime, I will read on my Kindle to dial down even further, but nothing of a business or creative nature. I prefer biographies and stories about real people – everything that can have gone right or wrong has already done so for somebody somewhere. It's not like we need to re-create the wheel; we just need to look, listen and learn. Kinda like we did in Pioppi.

I still sleep like a teenager, for fully eight hours or more, directing my crazy dreams in full Technicolor before waking up to the realization that there's no such thing as a bad day out there. If you ever get to visit Pioppi and take a seat in the morning sun outside that espresso bar in the centre of the village, you'll see they don't either! I can't wait to go back there.

My own rules are pretty straightforward: if I'm cooking or eating, there will always be good-quality, locally pro-duced extra virgin olive oil in the mix. We spend our money on quality protein so, when it comes to meat, eggs and fish, we stick to local, pasture-raised and wild where possible. As it is with food, so it is with red wine and coffee – I enjoy good-quality, local options. Fortunately, with its abundance of very high-quality local produce (including raw and fermented dairy), Cape Town allows me to tick all the right boxes and, relatively speaking, it is also very affordable. I make my own coconut butter, using raw coconut flesh, or cacaonut bombs, using a Nutribullet, so there is always a high-quality snack option to go with my coffee. As I'm a creature of habit, my food doesn't vary enormously week to week. Instead, I focus on the quality of the produce (including lots of vegetables and berries), on keeping things simple and on listening to my body. If I'm lifting, sprinting or HIITing, I will eat some extra carbs to support that intensity. Travelling long haul is something I do several times a year and, for many years now, I have fasted on planes. The body is more aggressively disrupted by food at weird times than by traversing time zones, something the science is now catching up to.

Here's a typical food week for me.

	Monday	Tuesday	Wednesday
Breakfast	No breakfast; only coffee with coconut cream	No breakfast; only coffee with coconut cream	No breakfast; only coffee with coconut cream
Brunch	2- or 3-egg mushroom omelette. Coffee with coconut cream. **Afternoon snack:** Tinned oysters; full-fat Greek yogurt with berries, a handful of nuts and cinnamon	Halloumi and fried tomato; vegetable soup made using chicken-bone broth; a small portion of oily fish (anchovies, sardines, pilchards); coffee with coconut cream	Full-fat Greek yogurt mixed with coconut cream and berries with a handful of nuts, a sprinkle of cinnamon and a pinch of turmeric; coffee with coconut cream **Afternoon snack:** Bacon nut-butter sliders – crispy, grilled bacon strips, topped generously with almond butter and a sprinkle of raw cacao
Dinner	Picanha steak (a superb Brazilian cut) served with creamed spinach and avocado side salad; 2 squares of dark chocolate (95 per cent cocoa solids), a cup of Earl Grey tea	Grilled salmon fillet with vegetables and sauerkraut; 2 squares of dark chocolate (95 per cent cocoa solids), a cup of Earl Grey tea	Grilled lamb chops with lots of mixed vegetables and side salad; 2 squares of dark chocolate (95 per cent cocoa solids), a cup of Earl Grey tea

Thursday	Friday	Saturday	Sunday
2 or 3 eggs any style, with smoked salmon and avocado; coffee with coconut cream	Bacon and 2 or 3 eggs, any style, with avocado (optional); coffee with coconut cream	Nut butter omelette; berries and full-fat Greek yogurt; coffee with coconut cream	Smoked salmon with 3 scrambled eggs on very high-quality sourdough (the only bread I eat, thanks to the fermentation process and the taste), avocado and crème fraiche; coffee with coconut cream
Smoothie with kefir and/or coconut milk, berries, a handful of nuts, some avocado with a tablespoon of coconut oil, a sprinkle of ground cinnamon, turmeric and fresh mint	Fish soup (made using chicken broth)	Greek-style salad	Smoothie, as before
Chicken-bone broth to start, with 1 tablespoon of extra virgin olive oil and salt to taste, followed by fresh pan-fried hake and vegetables; cacaonut bombs, a cup of Earl Grey tea	Low-carb pizza (and an honorable mention here of Chalk & Cork in Cape Town – they do it better than anyone!); cacaonut bombs, a cup of Earl Grey tea	Roast chicken with sweet potato and mixed vegetables; cacaonut bombs, a cup of Earl Grey tea	Baked trout with mixed vegetables; berries, nuts and cream

18.

Recommended Shopping List

*in moderation   # try to go organic

Pantry

apple cider vinegar (unfiltered)
chocolate (85 per cent-plus cocoa solids)
cinnamon
cocoa
coconut flakes
coconut flour
coconut milk
coconut oil
cumin
extra virgin olive oil
mustard seeds
nut butter*
nutmeg
nuts*
pepper
psyllium husk

pumpkin seeds
salt
sunflower seeds
turmeric

coffee
kombucha*
red wine*
sparkling water
tea

Clean meat

(preferably ethically sourced, with zero spices/additives/
sauces)

beef
bone broth
chicken
lamb
organ meat/bone marrow
pork

Dairy and fermented foods

butter from grass-fed cows*
crème fraîche*

feta cheese*
full-fat cheese*
full-fat cream/raw milk*
full-fat Greek yogurt
goat's cheese*
halloumi cheese*
kefir
sauerkraut/kimchi

Fish

(wild, locally caught and oily are best)

anchovies
cod
mackerel
monkfish
pilchards
salmon
sardines
shellfish
trout
tuna

Fresh produce

(local and organic, wherever possible)

basil
chillies#
coriander
eggs
garlic
ginger
mint
rosemary/other herbs

any leafy greens#
asparagus
aubergine
avocados
berries#
broccoli
Brussels sprouts
cabbage
cauliflower
celery#
cherries#
courgettes
cucumber#
fennel
green beans
lemons

mushrooms#
olives
onions
pumpkin*
rocket/leaves#
spinach/swiss chard/kale#
squash
sweet potatoes*
tomatoes#

PART THREE
Recipes

19.

Recipes

Breakfasts

Three-Egg Omelettes: Cheese and Spinach; Crab and Ricotta; Spicy
Peppers and Onions

Nut Butter Omelette

Baked Eggs – Turkish Style

Mexican Scrambled Eggs with Tomato Chilli Salsa

Boiled Eggs with Asparagus and Bacon Soldiers

Baked Avocado Egg Boats with Roast Cherry Tomatoes and Basil and
Chilli Oil

Greek Yogurt with Berries, Nuts and Seeds

Seedy Crackers with Smoked Salmon and Avocado

Coconut Pancakes

Warm Cinnamon Muesli with Berries

Chocolate Coconut Porridge with Poached Cherries

Sweet Potato Rösti with Poached Eggs and Harissa Crème Fraîche

Cauliflower Hash Browns with Goat's Cheese, Crispy Bacon and
Tomatoes

Lunches

Vegetable Frittata with Griddled Chicory

Crab and Saffron Frittata with Green Bean Salad

Greek Salad

Roast Vegetables, Labneh, Pomegranate and Walnut Salad

Tuna Niçoise

Thyme Roasted Chicken Caesar Salad

Lentil and Baked Goat's Cheese Salad with Tomato Dressing

Grilled Halloumi and Kale Salad with Tahini Yogurt Dressing

Minestrone made with Bone Broth

Chilled Cucumber and Avocado Soup

Prosciutto, Burrata and Tomato Salad with Basil Dressing

Smoked Mackerel Pâté, Bagna Cauda and Crudités

Monkfish Skewers with Basil Pesto

Courgetti Vongole

Karahi Prawns

Mediterranean Fish with Vegetable Hash and Aioli

Whole Roast Salmon with Lemon Herby Stuffing

Cauliflower Steaks with Feta

Cauliflower Cheese with Crispy Shallots

Slow-cooked Black Dal with Homemade Paneer and Charred Broccoli

Dad's Dal

Dinners

Cheese Burgers

Steak with Béarnaise Sauce and Griddled Broccoli

Meatballs in a Roast Tomato and Garlic Sauce with Sweet Potato Noodles

Cottage Pie with Cauliflower Mash

Harissa Lamb Chops

Karahi Lamb

Lamb Stew

Pulled Pork and Crackling Lettuce Wraps

Korean Stir-fried Pork Belly with Broccoli Kimchi Rice

Pork Chops with Sage Butter

Tandoori Masala Salmon with Raita

Spicy Salmon Curry

Thai-style Mussels and King Prawns

Pan-fried Cod with Clams

Pan-fried Mackerel with Kimchi

Monkfish Curry

Pan-fried Scallops with Cauliflower Mash and Griddled Leeks

Grandma's North Indian Chicken Curry

Chicken Schnitzel with Sauerkraut

Spatchcocked Chicken with Spiced Yogurt Marinade

Jerk Chicken Cauliflower Pizza

Roast Aubergines with Feta, Herbs and Yogurt Dressing

Pumpkin, Mushroom and Sage Butter Courgetti

Vegetable Curry

Low-carb Courgette Pizzas

Sides

Green Salad

Mixed Bean Salad

Mixed Green Vegetables

Broad Beans and Parmesan

Quick Kimchi

Cabbage Slaw

Quick Pickles

Vegetable Rice

Pancetta Brussels Sprouts with Whole Almonds

Punjabi Salad

Indian-style Mixed Vegetables

Tray-baked Roast Vegetables

Leek and Courgette Gratin

Cabbage Thoran

Breakfasts

Three-Egg Omelettes: Cheese and Spinach

SERVES 2

6 eggs

¼ of a nutmeg, grated

sea salt and freshly ground black pepper

20g butter

150g baby spinach

2 tablespoons extra virgin olive oil

100g Cheddar cheese, grated

1 avocado, destoned and sliced, to serve

Crack the eggs into a jug and beat thoroughly. Add the nutmeg and season with salt and pepper.

Put 10g of the butter into a frying pan over a low heat. Add the spinach to the pan and cook for a couple of minutes until wilted, then remove from the heat and divide in two, discarding any liquid left in the pan.

Put half the remaining butter and half the oil into the frying pan, over a low heat. Once the butter and oil stop foaming and start to smell nutty, add half the egg mixture and half the spinach. Using a wooden spoon, gently move the eggs around, pulling in the set edges and redistributing the uncooked egg, covering the base of the pan, until the omelette is half cooked. Add half the grated Cheddar.

Once the omelette looks very nearly cooked and the cheese has begun to melt, carefully slide the omelette on to a plate. Repeat with the remaining ingredients.

Serve immediately, with the avocado.

Crab and Ricotta

SERVES 2

6 eggs

100g crab meat, white and brown (tinned or fresh)

80g ricotta

10g finely chopped fresh chives

sea salt and freshly ground black pepper

10g butter

2 tablespoons extra virgin olive oil

1 avocado, destoned and sliced, to serve

Crack the eggs into a jug and beat thoroughly. Add the crab meat, ricotta and chives and mix well. Season with salt and pepper.

Put half the butter and half the oil into a frying pan over a low heat. Once the butter and oil stop foaming and start to smell nutty, add half the egg mixture. Using a wooden spoon, gently move the eggs around, pulling in the set edges and redistributing the uncooked egg, covering the base of the pan.

Once the omelette looks very nearly cooked, carefully slide it on to a plate. Repeat with the remaining ingredients.

Serve immediately, with the avocado.

Spicy Peppers and Onions

SERVES 2

6 eggs
½ teaspoon hot smoked paprika
½ teaspoon cayenne pepper
1 teaspoon chilli flakes
sea salt and freshly ground black pepper
10g butter
2 tablespoons extra virgin olive oil

½ a red pepper, diced
½ a green pepper, diced
½ a yellow pepper, diced
1 white onion, diced
80g Manchego cheese, grated (Cheddar would also work well)
1 avocado, destoned and sliced, to serve

Crack the eggs into a jug and beat thoroughly. Mix in the spices and season with salt and pepper.

Put the butter and the oil into the frying pan over a low heat. Once the butter and oil stop foaming and start to smell nutty, add the peppers and the onion. Cook for 5 to 6 minutes, stirring occasionally, until the peppers start to soften and the onion turns a light golden brown.

Add the egg mixture and, using a wooden spoon, gently move the eggs around, incorporating the peppers and onion. Pull in the set edges and redistribute the uncooked egg, keeping the base of the pan covered. Add half the grated cheese.

Once the omelette looks very nearly cooked and the cheese has begun to melt, carefully slide the omelette on to a plate. Repeat with the remaining ingredients.

Serve immediately, with the avocado.

Nut Butter Omelette

SERVES 2

6 eggs

120g nut butter (almond, cashew, peanut, hazelnut, macadamia, etc)

1 teaspoon cinnamon, or to taste

1 teaspoon vanilla extract

½ teaspoon turmeric

2 teaspoons coconut oil

4 tablespoons natural yogurt and 100g mixed berries, to serve

Put all the ingredients apart from the coconut oil, yogurt and berries into a food processor (or use a stick blender in a jug) and blitz until well mixed and frothy.

Melt half the oil in a frying pan over a low heat, swirl the pan to cover the base and pour in half the omelette mixture. Again, swirl the pan to cover the base. Cook for 4 to 5 minutes. This has a different texture from that of a normal omelette, more like a pancake.

Carefully slide the omelette on to a plate. Repeat with the remaining ingredients.

To serve, cover with the yogurt, fresh berries and, if desired, an extra sprinkle of cinnamon.

·

Mexican scrambled eggs with tomato chilli salsa

·

Boiled eggs with asparagus and bacon soldiers

·

Seedy crackers with smoked salmon and avocado

·

Chocolate coconut porridge with poached cherries

·

Sweet potato rösti with poached eggs and harissa crème fraîche

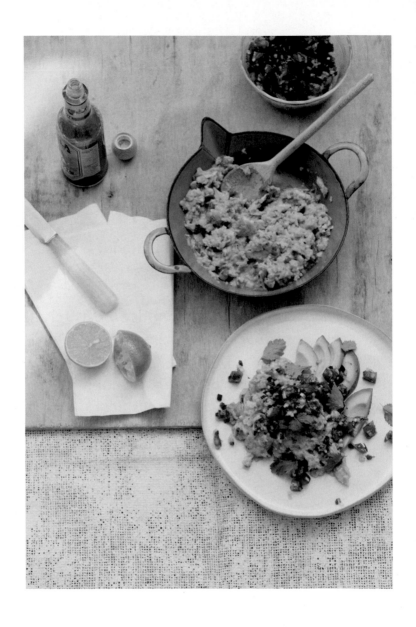

**Mexican scrambled eggs with
tomato chilli salsa**

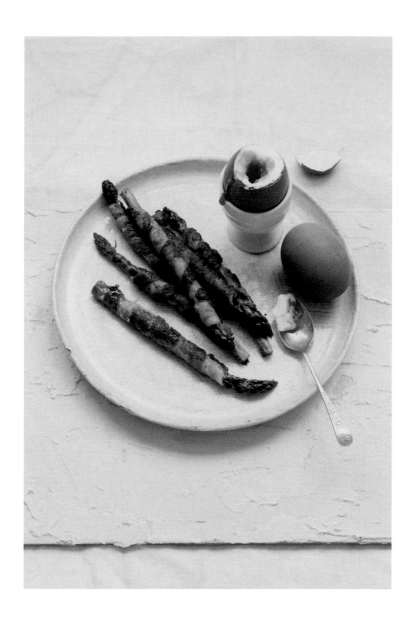

**Boiled eggs with asparagus
and bacon soldiers**

BREAKFAST

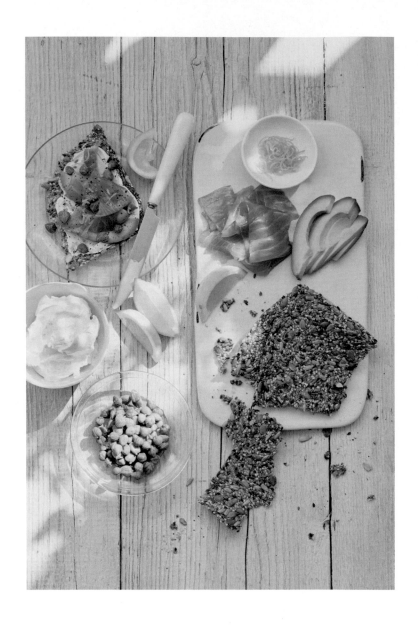

**Seedy crackers with smoked salmon
and avocado**

BREAKFAST

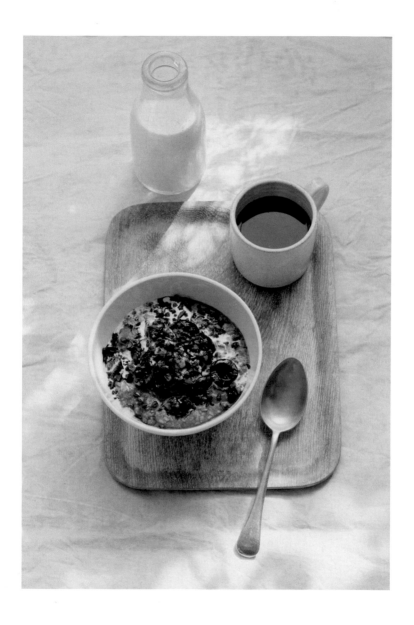

**Chocolate coconut porridge with
poached cherries**

BREAKFAST

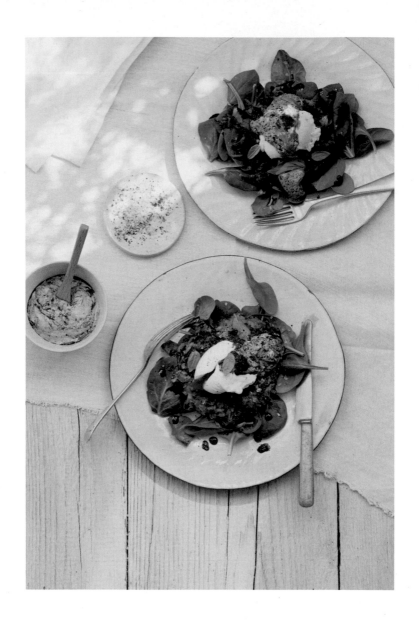

**Sweet potato rösti with poached eggs
and harissa crème fraîche**

BREAKFAST

·

Vegetable frittata with griddled chicory

·

Roast vegetables, labneh, pomegranate and walnut salad

·

Thyme roasted chicken Caesar salad

·

Grilled halloumi and kale salad with tahini yogurt dressing

·

Chilled cucumber and avocado soup

·

Monkfish skewers with basil pesto

·

Cauliflower steaks with feta

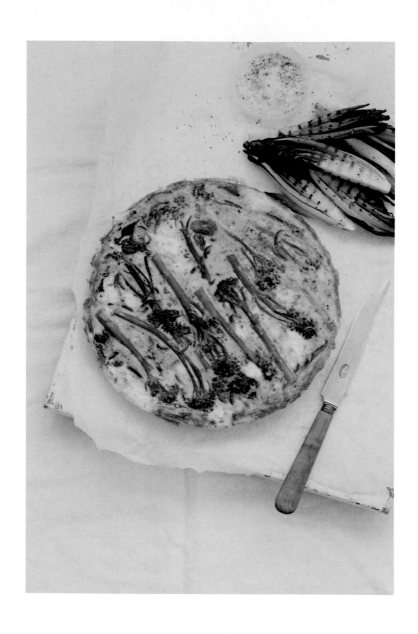

Vegetable frittata with griddled chicory

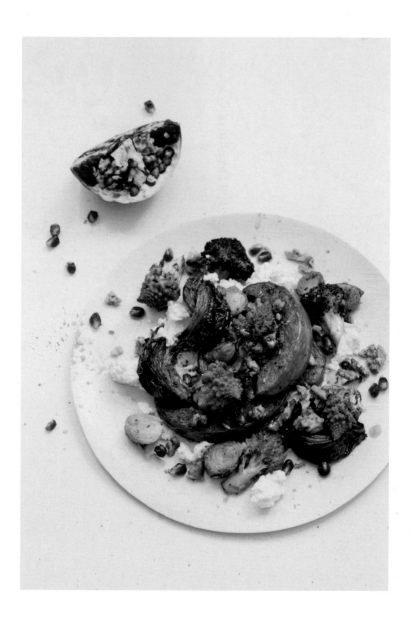

**Roast vegetables, labneh, pomegranate
and walnut salad**

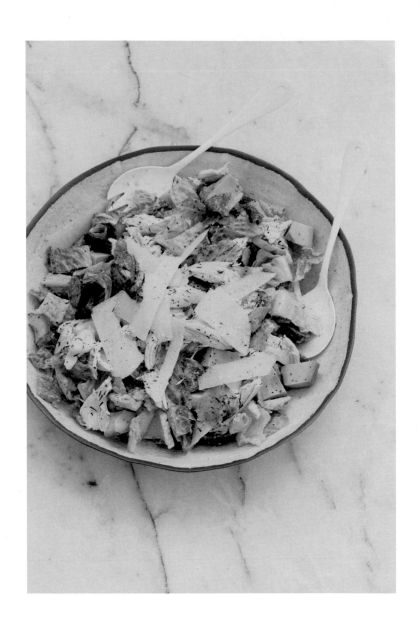

Thyme roasted chicken Caesar salad

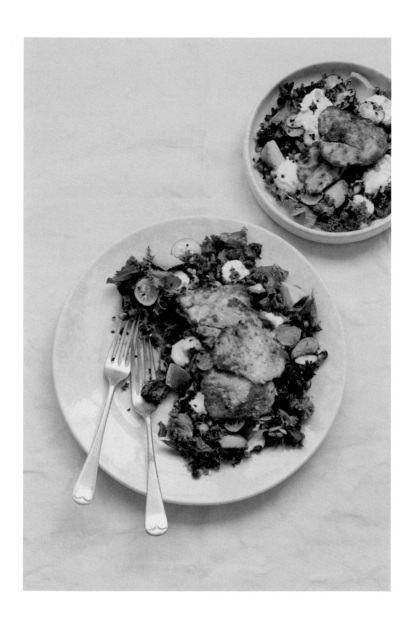

Grilled halloumi and kale salad with tahini yogurt dressing

LUNCH

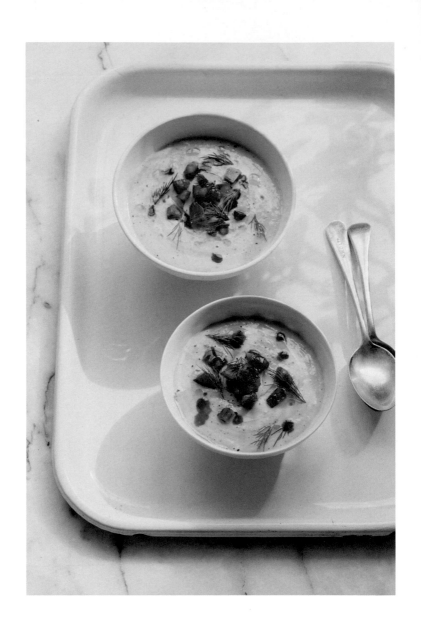

Chilled cucumber and avocado soup

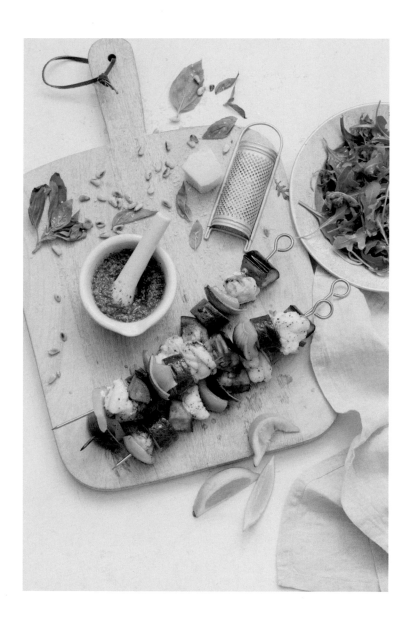

Monkfish skewers with basil pesto

LUNCH

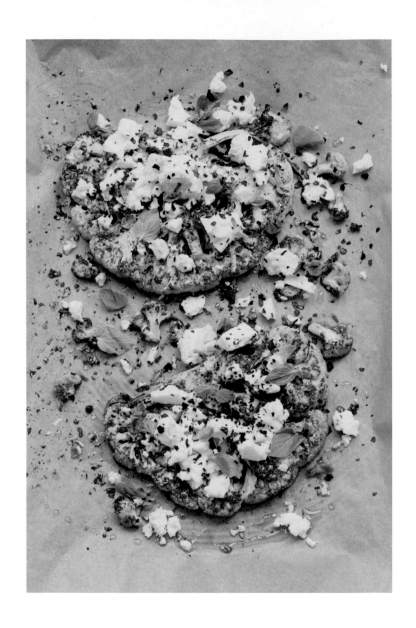

Cauliflower steaks with feta

·

Cheese burgers

·

Meatballs in a roast tomato and garlic sauce with sweet potato noodles

·

Pork chops with sage butter

·

Tandoori masala salmon with raita

·

Pan-fried mackerel with kimchi

·

Spatchcocked chicken with spiced yogurt marinade

·

Jerk chicken cauliflower pizza

·

Roast aubergines with feta, herbs and yogurt dressing

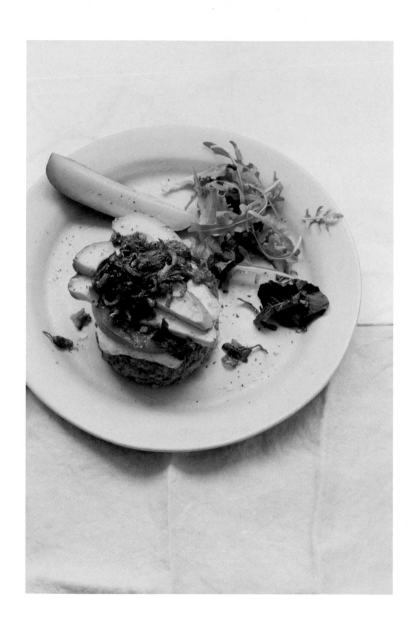

Cheese burgers

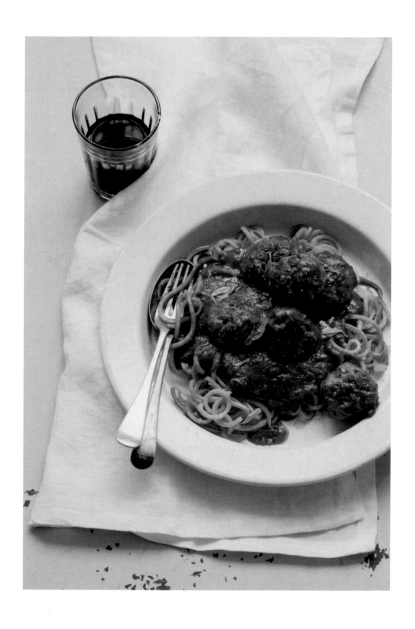

**Meatballs in a roast tomato and garlic
sauce with sweet potato noodles**

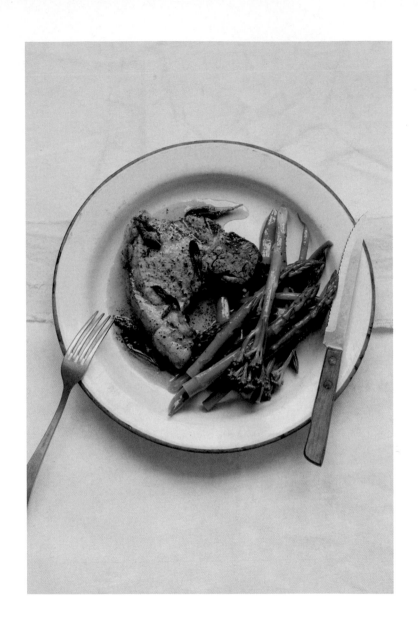

Pork chops with sage butter

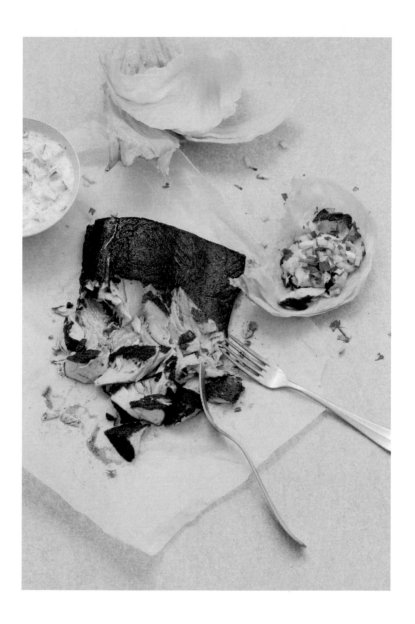

Tandoori masala salmon with raita

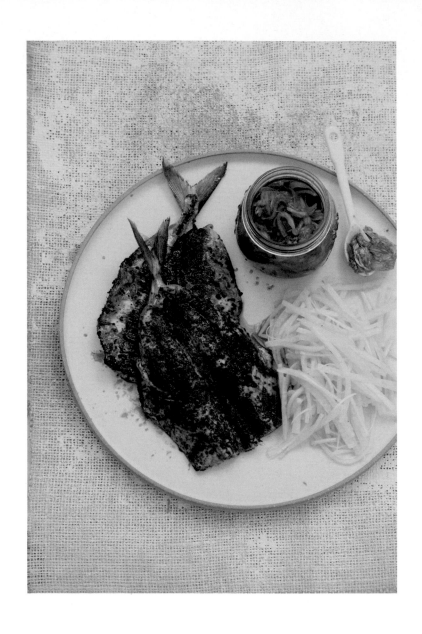

Pan-fried mackerel with kimchi

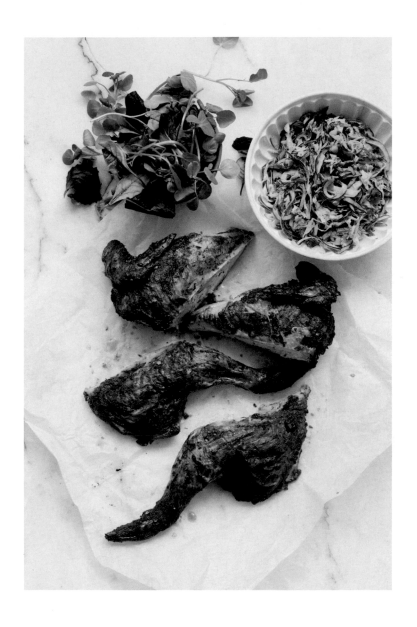

Spatchcocked chicken with spiced yogurt marinade

DINNER

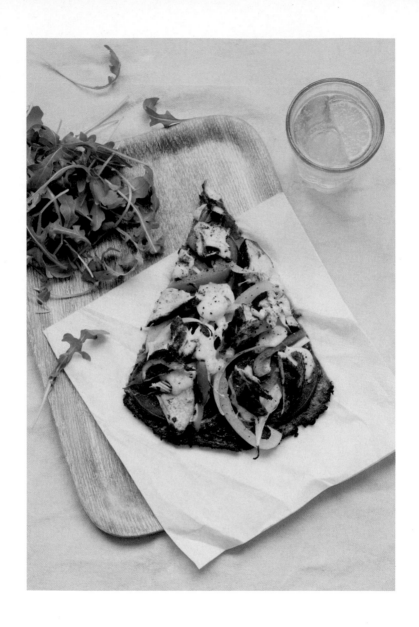

Jerk chicken cauliflower pizza

DINNER

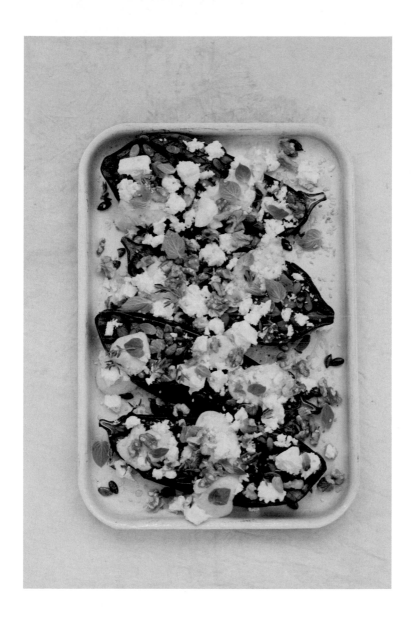

**Roast aubergines with feta, herbs
and yogurt dressing**

DINNER

Baked Eggs – Turkish Style

SERVES 2

2 tablespoons extra virgin olive oil

a knob of butter

1 green pepper, diced

1 onion, chopped

2 teaspoons pul biber (or paprika)

1 teaspoon ground cumin

1 teaspoon dried oregano

1 tablespoon tomato purée

3 cloves of garlic, finely grated

1 x 400g tin of good-quality plum tomatoes

100g baby spinach

4 eggs

4 tablespoons natural yogurt, 2 tablespoons extra virgin olive oil, 1 tablespoon nigella seeds and a handful of fresh coriander leaves, to serve

Put the oil and the butter into a wide-based sauté pan, over a medium heat. When the butter has melted, add the green pepper and the onion. Cook for 5 minutes until they start to soften. Add the cumin and oregano and mix well. Cook for a further 2 minutes.

Add the tomato purée and garlic and stir to coat the pepper and onion. Cook for 90 seconds, stirring continuously, as the purée can easily over-caramelize and the garlic can become bitter.

Add the chopped tomatoes. Half-fill the tin with water, swish, and add to the pan. Stir everything together, reduce the heat and leave to simmer for 15 minutes, stirring halfway through.

When the sauce begins to thicken, add the spinach and stir through until it starts to wilt.

Make four wells in the mixture and crack an egg into each. Bake in the heat of the juicy tomato mixture for 10 to 12 minutes, or until the whites become opaque.

To serve, spoon on the yogurt, drizzle with extra virgin olive oil and scatter with the nigella seeds and coriander leaves.

Mexican Scrambled Eggs with Tomato Chilli Salsa

SERVES 2

FOR THE TOMATO CHILLI SALSA:

4 ripe tomatoes, deseeded and chopped into 5mm dice

1 banana shallot, finely chopped

2 red chillies, finely chopped; deseeded, if preferred

1 clove of garlic, finely grated

10g chopped fresh coriander

2 tablespoons extra virgin olive oil

1 lime, juice only

sea salt and freshly ground black pepper

FOR THE SCRAMBLED EGGS:

10g butter

1 tablespoon extra virgin olive oil

4 spring onions, thinly sliced

2 jalapeño chillies, finely chopped

4 eggs

sea salt and freshly ground black pepper

1 avocado, destoned and thinly sliced, a handful of fresh coriander, chopped, and (optional) some hot sauce (Cholula, for example), to serve

Start by making the tomato chilli salsa, to give the flavours time to mingle. Place all the ingredients, other than the lime juice, in a mixing bowl and stir well, but gently, taking care not to break down the tomatoes too much. Add the lime juice, and season with salt and pepper.

Now make the scrambled eggs. Put the butter and oil into a frying pan, over a medium heat. Once the butter has melted and starts to smell nutty, turn the heat down and add the spring onions and chillies. Cook for 2 to 3 minutes.

While it's cooking, crack the eggs into a jug and beat thoroughly.

Season with salt and pepper. Add the spring onions and chillies, moving the eggs around with a wooden spoon to scramble them.

To serve, divide the avocado, eggs and tomato salsa between two plates. Scatter with the coriander leaves and add a dash of hot sauce, if you like an extra kick.

Boiled Eggs with Asparagus and Bacon Soldiers

SERVES 2

12 asparagus spears

12 rashers smoked streaky bacon

10g butter

1 tablespoon extra virgin olive oil

4 large eggs, at room temperature

sea salt and freshly ground black pepper

Take one rasher of bacon and one asparagus spear and, starting at one end, tightly wrap the bacon around the asparagus. Repeat until you have all the spears assembled.

Place the butter and oil in a frying pan large enough to hold all the asparagus at once. When the butter has melted, add the prepared asparagus. Bring a saucepan of water to the boil.

Carefully lower the eggs into the boiling water with a slotted spoon. If you like a really soft, dippy egg, cook for 5½ to 6 minutes. If you like your eggs a little harder, cook for a further minute or two. (Remember, they will become hard-boiled if cooked for 9 to 10 minutes.)

While the eggs are cooking, turn the asparagus spears every couple of minutes until they are an even golden brown. Season with salt and pepper.

Divide between two plates and serve.

Baked Avocado Egg Boats with Roast Cherry Tomatoes and Basil and Chilli Oil

SERVES 2

FOR THE BASIL AND CHILLI OIL:

4 tablespoons extra virgin olive oil

10g finely chopped fresh basil leaves

1 red chilli, very finely chopped

FOR THE ROAST CHERRY TOMATOES:

3 sprigs of thyme

1 clove of garlic, sliced

2 stems cherry tomatoes, on the vine

a drizzle of extra virgin olive oil

sea salt and freshly ground black pepper

FOR THE AVOCADO EGG BOATS:

2 avocados, halved and destoned

1 teaspoon extra virgin olive oil

4 medium-sized eggs

1 small cooking chorizo, finely diced

sea salt and freshly ground black pepper

5g chopped fresh flat-leaf parsley

Preheat the oven to 180°C/160°C fan. Next, make the chilli oil, to enable the flavours to blend. Place the olive oil in a small bowl, add the basil and the chilli, mix well and set to one side.

Line a baking tray with greaseproof paper and lay the thyme and garlic on it, to make a bed for the tomatoes. Place the tomatoes on top and drizzle with olive oil. Season with salt and pepper. Cook in the oven for 20 to 25 minutes.

Line an ovenproof dish that will hold the avocado halves snugly with baking paper. (Alternatively, make stands for the avocado halves to sit on from tin foil, to prevent them tipping over.)

Place the avocado halves in the dish. Brush the olive oil over the flesh of the avocados. Crack an egg into a ramekin, then scoop up the yolk with a spoon and drop it into the hole of an avocado half. Top up with as much egg white as will fit. (Depending on the size of the stone, you may need to scoop out a little of the flesh to make room for the egg.) Repeat three times. Sprinkle with the diced chorizo, season with salt and pepper and cook on the middle shelf of the oven for 8 to 10 minutes.

To serve, divide the avocados between two plates and drizzle with any juices from the pan. Place a vine of tomatoes alongside, drizzle with basil and chilli oil and scatter with parsley.

Greek Yogurt with Berries, Nuts and Seeds

SERVES 2

20g walnuts	10g sunflower seeds
20g flaked almonds	10g pumpkin seeds
20g blanched hazelnuts	10g golden flaxseeds
300ml Greek yogurt	10g brown flaxseeds
60g raspberries	
60g blueberries	
60g strawberries, hulled and halved	

Preheat the oven to 140°C/120° fan.

Place all the nuts on a baking sheet and cook for 12 to 15 minutes, stirring and shaking halfway through, until they take on a light golden colour. Remove from the oven and allow to cool.

To serve, divide the yogurt, berries, nuts and seeds between two bowls.

Seedy Crackers with Smoked Salmon and Avocado

SERVES 2

60g cream cheese

1 lemon, zest and juice

½ an avocado, destoned and sliced,

100g smoked salmon

50g capers

freshly ground black pepper

30g sesame seeds

30g golden flaxseeds

30g brown flaxseeds

15g poppy seeds

2 tablespoons psyllium husks

a pinch of sea salt

180ml cold water

FOR THE SEEDY CRACKERS:

30g sunflower seeds

30g pumpkin seeds

This will make more crackers than you need for one meal, but you can keep them in an airtight container for at least a week.

Preheat the oven to 160°C/140°C fan. Line a baking tray with non-stick baking paper.

Place all the dry ingredients for the crackers in a mixing bowl and mix well. Add the water and stir, to bring the mixture together. Set to one side for approximately 20 minutes so the seeds absorb the water.

Once the mixture is thick, like wallpaper paste, tip it on to the baking tray and, using a palette knife, spread the mixture out as thinly as you can, without making any holes.

Place in the oven for 1 hour, rotating the tray 180 degrees halfway through. When cooked, the mixture should have fully dried out, have the appearance of a cracker, be golden in colour and smell of toasted seeds. If not, cook for a further 10 minutes, then check again. Repeat, if necessary. Remove from the oven and leave to cool, then carefully peel the mixture off the baking paper and snap into rustic crackers.

Tip the cream cheese into a small bowl and finely grate in the lemon zest. Mix well.

To serve, spread the cracker with the lemony cream cheese, add a slice of avocado and top with some smoked salmon, a few capers, a squeeze of lemon juice and a twist of black pepper.

Coconut Pancakes

SERVES 2

FOR THE COCONUT PANCAKES:

150g coconut flour, sieved

½ teaspoon baking powder

4 eggs

1 teaspoon ground cinnamon

½ teaspoon vanilla extract

FOR THE TOPPING:

4 tablespoons natural yogurt

80g blueberries

80g cherries, destoned and halved

30g pecan nuts

30g coconut flakes, toasted

6 teaspoons coconut oil, for frying

Place all the pancake ingredients in a mixing bowl and blend into a batter, using an electric whisk. This should only take a minute or two.

Melt 2 teaspoons of the oil into a large frying pan on a high heat. When the pan is hot, drop in 2 heaped tablespoons of the pancake batter, to make two pancakes – each should be the size of a Scotch pancake. When the top starts to dry out, after 2 to 3 minutes, flip the pancake. Be careful: they are less robust than pancakes made with flour.

Cook the pancakes for another 2 minutes, then transfer to a plate. Repeat until you have used up all the batter. (There should be enough batter for three pancakes per person.)

To serve, stack the pancakes, pour over the yogurt and scatter with the fruit, pecans and coconut flakes.

Warm Cinnamon Muesli with Berries

SERVES 2

FOR THE MUESLI:

50g jumbo rolled oats

30g blanched hazelnuts

30g walnuts

30g blanched almonds

20g poppy seeds

20g brown flaxseeds

20g sunflower seeds

2 teaspoons ground cinnamon

50g coconut oil, melted

FOR THE TOPPING:

200ml coconut cream

150g blackberries

150g raspberries

2 tablespoons ground golden
flaxseeds, to serve

Preheat the oven to 170°C/150°C fan. Line a large lipped baking tray with non-stick baking paper. Tip all the muesli ingredients on to it and mix well, making sure that everything is coated with the coconut oil and cinnamon.

Place in the oven for 10 minutes, then stir. Return to the oven for another 10 minutes, stir again, then return to the oven for a further 10 minutes.

While the muesli is baking, put the coconut cream into a small saucepan and place on a low heat. Once it's warm, add the fruit and poach for 10 minutes.

To serve, divide the muesli between two bowls, pour over the fruity coconut cream and sprinkle with the golden flaxseeds.

Chocolate Coconut Porridge with Poached Cherries

SERVES 2

FOR THE POACHED CHERRIES:

160g cherries, destoned and halved

½ a vanilla pod, split

100ml water

FOR THE PORRIDGE:

80g coconut flour

60g desiccated coconut

40g coconut flakes

2 tablespoons raw cacao powder

300ml coconut milk

50ml double cream and 2 tablespoons grated 85% dark chocolate or 20g cacao nibs, to serve

Place the cherries, vanilla pod and water in a small saucepan and put over a low heat for 20 minutes. The poaching process should be gradual so the fruit releases its natural sugars and juices.

While the fruit is poaching, put all the porridge ingredients into a medium-sized saucepan and place over a low heat. Gently cook for 10 to 15 minutes, stirring regularly, until the porridge starts to thicken and become creamy. Continue until the porridge has reached your preferred consistency.

To serve, divide the porridge between two bowls, add the fruit and syrup, drizzle with cream and top with grated chocolate or cacao nibs.

Sweet Potato Rösti with Poached Eggs and Harissa Crème Fraîche

SERVES 2

FOR THE RÖSTI:

2 sweet potatoes, peeled

40g butter

4 tablespoons extra virgin olive oil

1 medium onion, very finely chopped

2 cloves of garlic, finely grated

10g chopped fresh basil leaves

1 egg, lightly beaten

sea salt and freshly ground black pepper

FOR THE POACHED EGGS:

50ml white wine vinegar

2 large eggs

FOR THE HARISSA CRÈME FRAÎCHE

150ml crème fraîche

2 tablespoons rose harissa

100g baby spinach and basil leaves, to serve

Grate the sweet potatoes, place on a clean tea towel, pull up the corners and wring out firmly over the sink to get rid of any excess liquid. Place the grated sweet potatoes into a large mixing bowl.

Put half the butter and half the oil into a medium-sized frying pan, over a low heat, add the onion and gently fry. After about 5 minutes, add the garlic and cook for another minute. Tip into the bowl with the grated sweet potato. Add the basil and the egg and mix together. Season with salt and pepper, divide in half and shape with your hands into two circles.

Put the remaining butter and oil into the frying pan, over a low heat. Add the röstis and press down gently. Cook for approximately 10 minutes, checking occasionally that the base isn't burning, then flip and cook for another 10 minutes. If they look a little dry, or look as if they might stick, put a few tiny knobs of butter around the röstis.

Using the tip of a sharp knife, check to see if the röstis are cooked through. If not, cook for a few more minutes then check again.

While the röstis are cooking, bring a large saucepanful of water to simmering point. Add the vinegar. Crack the eggs into separate ramekins. Stir the water to create a vortex, slowly drop one egg at the side of the pan and repeat with the second. The eggs should be swept neatly into the middle of the pan. If you like a runny egg, cook for 3 minutes, or, if you prefer a firm yolk, up to 7. When the eggs are done, lift out of the water with a slotted spoon and drain on kitchen paper.

In a small bowl, mix together the crème fraîche and the harissa.

To serve, place half the spinach on each plate as a bed. Top with a rösti, a poached egg, a good dollop of the harissa crème fraiche and a few basil leaves, and season to taste.

Cauliflower Hash Browns with Goat's Cheese, Crispy Bacon and Tomatoes

SERVES 2

FOR THE HASH BROWNS:

½ a cauliflower, cut into florets

1 onion, finely chopped

1 large egg and 1 yolk, lightly beaten

1 tablespoon Dijon mustard

10g finely chopped fresh chives,

sea salt and freshly ground black pepper

20g butter

4 tablespoons extra virgin olive oil

100g goat's cheese, 8 rashers unsmoked streaky bacon, 2 beef tomatoes, sliced, and a dab of Dijon mustard, to serve

Preheat the oven to 190°C/170°C fan.

Place the cauliflower florets in the bowl of a food processor and pulse a few times to make even-sized crumbs – a bit chunkier than breadcrumbs. Put into a clean tea towel, pull in the corners and wring out firmly over the sink to remove any excess liquid.

Tip the cauliflower into a large mixing bowl. Add all the other ingredients for the hash browns, except for the butter and oil, and mix well.

Line a baking sheet with non-stick baking paper and tip the hash brown mixture, on to it. Using a small ring mould, cut six circles, pressing the mixture down firmly into the ring each time so it will stick together, then gently sliding the mould off. Place the baking sheet in the oven. Cook for 20 minutes, then remove from the oven, top each hash brown with a couple of slices of goat's cheese and return to the oven for 5 minutes. After this, turn the oven off but leave the tray in to keep warm.

While the hash browns are finishing, put the bacon rashers into a frying pan and cook until crispy, turning occasionally, then place on the baking tray in the oven with the hash browns.

Using the same pan, turn up the heat and fry the beef tomatoes in the bacon fat for 2 to 3 minutes, then flip and fry the other side, seasoning with salt and pepper.

To serve, divide the hash browns between two plates and top with the bacon and tomatoes. Drizzle with any remaining pan juices, season with some fresh pepper and add a dollop of mustard on the side.

Lunches

Vegetable Frittata with Griddled Chicory

SERVES 6 TO 8

FOR THE VEGETABLE FRITTATA:

8 large eggs

100ml double cream

½ teaspoon dried oregano

½ a nutmeg, grated

sea salt and freshly ground black pepper

10g butter

2 tablespoons extra virgin olive oil

1 red onion, thinly sliced

150g chestnut mushrooms, sliced

60g kale, torn into pieces

80g tenderstem broccoli

100g feta cheese, crumbled

FOR THE GRIDDLED CHICORY:

4 heads of red chicory, quartered

2 tablespoons extra virgin olive oil

sea salt and freshly ground black pepper

2 tablespoons hazelnuts, toasted and roughly chopped, to serve

Crack the eggs into a jug and lightly whisk. Add the double cream, oregano and nutmeg, and season with salt and pepper. Whisk together and put to one side.

Put the butter and oil into a 26cm frying pan, with a handle that can go under the grill, on a medium heat. Once the butter has melted, add the onion. Cook until it starts to soften, then add the mushrooms, stirring continuously.

After 5 minutes, add the kale and the broccoli. Allow everything to cook together for another 5 minutes.

Turn the heat down and add the eggs. Mix them around the vegetables, moving the cooked edges in towards the middle of the pan and swirling the pan to redistribute the uncooked egg to fill the gaps. Add the feta and check that the vegetables are evenly distributed. Allow to cook undisturbed for 2 to 3 minutes, while you light the grill.

Once the grill is hot, place the frying pan underneath it for approximately 5 minutes to finish cooking the frittata. Shake the pan to check none of the egg wobbles. When it is set, remove from the heat and allow to cool in the pan for a few minutes, then slide it on to a plate or chopping board.

Heat a griddle pan, brush the cut sides of the chicory with oil, season lightly and place on the pan. Cook each side for 3 minutes. Do not worry if some of the leaves char; it will add a lovely bitter, smoky taste.

To serve, place a slice of the frittata on each plate, with two or three pieces of chicory, and scatter with the hazelnuts.

Crab and Saffron Frittata with Green Bean Salad
SERVES 6 TO 8

FOR THE FRITTATA:

8 large eggs

150ml double cream

sea salt and freshly ground
black pepper

a good pinch of saffron

20g butter

2 tablespoons extra virgin
olive oil

2 large leeks, finely sliced

1 teaspoon cayenne pepper

200g white crab meat (tinned
or fresh)

1 lemon, zest and juice

FOR THE GREEN BEAN SALAD:

200g green beans, topped
and tailed

200g mangetouts

2 tablespoons extra virgin
olive oil

1 tablespoon apple cider vinegar

sea salt and freshly ground
black pepper

50g flaked almonds

Crack the eggs into a jug and lightly whisk. Add the double cream and season with salt and pepper. Whisk together and put to one side.

Put the saffron into an egg cup, add 1 tablespoon of hot water and allow to infuse.

Put the butter and oil into a 26cm frying pan, with a handle that can go under the grill, on a medium heat. Once the butter has melted, add the leeks. Cook for approximately 10 minutes, until softened. Add the saffron in its liquid and the cayenne, and stir to coat the leeks and evaporate the water.

Add the crab meat and mix well, then add the lemon zest and a squeeze of lemon juice, stirring well.

Turn the heat right down and add the eggs. Stir the crab and leek into the egg mixture, moving the cooked edges in towards the middle of the pan and swirling the pan to redistribute any uncooked egg to fill the gaps. Allow to cook undisturbed for 2 to 3 minutes, while you light the grill.

When the grill is hot, place the frying pan underneath it for approximately 5 minutes to finish cooking the frittata. Shake the pan to check none of the egg wobbles. When it is set, remove from the heat and allow to cool in the pan for a few minutes, then slide it on to a plate or chopping board.

Put a little water into a pan and bring to the boil. Place a steamer in the pan. Add the beans and the mangetouts and steam for 5 minutes. While they are cooking, put the oil, vinegar and some salt and pepper into a mixing bowl and whisk together.

When the beans are done, tip them into the bowl, add the flaked almonds and toss to coat everything in the dressing.

To serve, place a slice of frittata on each plate and serve with the beans.

Greek Salad

SERVES 2

4 ripe tomatoes, on the vine, each
cut into 6 chunks

½ a cucumber, halved and sliced
on the diagonal

1 small red onion, halved and
thinly sliced

1 green pepper, deseeded and
roughly chopped

100g Kalamata olives (or other
black olives)

100g feta cheese, roughly
crumbled

FOR THE SALAD DRESSING:

3 tablespoons extra virgin
olive oil

1 tablespoon red wine vinegar

½ teaspoon dried oregano

½ teaspoon dried mint

sea salt and freshly ground
black pepper

a few fresh mint leaves and a
drizzle of extra virgin olive oil,
to serve

Super quick and easy to do, this salad is all about assembly. First of all,
put all the salad ingredients into a large mixing bowl.

In a small jug, whisk together all the ingredients for the dressing. Pour
the dressing over the salad and toss gently – you don't want the feta to
break down completely.

To serve, transfer to a bowl and add the fresh mint leaves and a drizzle
of extra virgin olive oil.

Roast Vegetables, Labneh, Pomegranate and Walnut Salad

You'll need to start the labneh the day before you want to eat this dish, but it really is worth the wait. You could buy ready-made labneh, however, or substitute with Greek yogurt.

SERVES 4

(This will make more than you need for this recipe but the rest will keep in the fridge for up to a week.)

FOR THE LABNEH:
500g natural yogurt
500g Greek yogurt
a pinch of salt

FOR THE ROAST VEGETABLES:
100g Brussels sprouts, halved
1 red onion, sliced into 8 wedges
6 cauliflower florets
6 broccoli florets

½ a small squash, cut into wedges
4 tablespoons extra virgin olive oil
1 tablespoon za'atar
sea salt and freshly ground black pepper
60g walnuts

½ a pomegranate, a drizzle of extra virgin olive oil and 5g fresh flat-leaf parsley, to serve

You will need: a large piece of muslin (approximately 60cm x 120cm)

For the labneh

Put both types of yogurt into a large bowl, add the salt and mix together.

Take the piece of muslin and fold in half. Lay this in a colander with the corners hanging evenly over the sides. Pour the yogurt into the middle then gather up the corners of the muslin and knot firmly together, leaving space to hang the parcel. Hook it over a kitchen cupboard handle, out of direct heat and sunlight, place a bowl underneath to catch the liquid and leave for approximately 12 hours.

When it is ready, discard the liquid and transfer the labneh, which should be firm and creamy, into an airtight container.

Preheat the oven to 210°C/190°C fan. Line a large roasting tray with baking paper and put all the vegetables into it. Add the olive oil, za'atar and some seasoning and mix with your hands to make sure all the vegetables are evenly covered.

Place in the oven for 30 minutes, turning halfway through.

Remove the tray from the oven and, using your hands, crush the walnuts over the vegetables and return to the oven for another 10 minutes. Keep an eye on it, as you don't want anything to burn at the last minute.

To serve, put 3 tablespoons of the labneh on each plate and spread out with the back of a spoon. Divide the vegetables and walnuts between the two plates. Hold the cut side of the pomegranate over the plate and, using a wooden spoon, bash the skin to release the seeds (a little bit messy but lots of fun). Add a drizzle of extra virgin olive oil and the fresh parsley leaves before diving in.

Tuna Niçoise

SERVES 2

FOR THE SALAD:

200g fresh tuna steak

1 teaspoon extra virgin olive oil

sea salt and freshly ground black pepper

3 large eggs, room temperature

100g green beans, topped and tailed

2 little gem lettuces, leaves torn into chunks

1 avocado, destoned and cut into cubes

100g cherry tomatoes, halved

½ a red onion, finely sliced

50g black olives

FOR THE DRESSING:

2 anchovy fillets, finely chopped

6 tablespoons extra virgin olive oil

2 tablespoons red wine vinegar

½ teaspoon mustard powder

1 clove of garlic, crushed to a paste

sea salt and freshly ground black pepper

Place a frying pan on a high heat. Rub the tuna steak with a little oil, salt and pepper and put into the pan when it's hot. Cook for 2 minutes each side – you want the tuna still to be pink in the middle like a medium-rare steak. Remove from the pan and leave to rest on a chopping board.

Bring a saucepan of water to the boil and, with a slotted spoon, gently lower the eggs into it. Cook for 7 minutes if you like a soft yolk, or add a minute (up to a maximum of 10) for a hard-boiled egg. When the eggs are done, run them under cold water to stop them cooking any further.

Bring the saucepan of water back up to the boil, with a steamer basket on top. Place the beans in the steamer for 4 to 5 minutes, until al dente.

Divide the little gem leaves, avocado, beans, tomatoes, onion and olives between two plates.

Peel the eggs and carefully slice in half. Give three halves to each person.

Slice the tuna into half-centimetre-thick slices and place on top.

Put all the ingredients for the salad dressing into a small, clean jam jar. Put the lid on the jar and shake well to blend. Pour over the salad, and enjoy.

Thyme Roasted Chicken Caesar Salad

SERVES 4 TO 6

FOR THE ROAST CHICKEN:

1 free-range chicken, 1.6kg approximate weight

2 tablespoons extra virgin olive oil

2 tablespoons dried wild thyme

sea salt and freshly ground black pepper

1 lemon, halved

2 bay leaves

1 bunch of fresh thyme

FOR THE CAESAR DRESSING:

1 egg yolk

1 clove of garlic, crushed to a paste

4 anchovy fillets in olive oil, crushed to a paste

½ teaspoon Dijon mustard

1 teaspoon water

150ml extra virgin olive oil

100ml natural yogurt

50g Parmesan cheese, finely grated

freshly ground black pepper

½ a lemon, juice only

FOR THE SALAD:

2–3 romaine heart lettuces, root removed, leaves separated

12 cherry tomatoes, halved

1 avocado, destoned and cut into chunks

Parmesan shavings

Preheat the oven to 210°C/190°C fan and line a large roasting tin with baking paper. Put the chicken into the pan and drizzle the oil over the breast and legs. Rub the dried thyme and some seasoning all over the chicken, covering the legs, wings and breast. Place the lemon halves, fresh thyme and bay leaves in the cavity. Place the tray in the oven and cook for 1 hour (or until the flesh is opaque and, when a knife is inserted into the thickest part of the leg, the juices run clear), turning the roasting tin halfway through. Remove from the oven and leave to rest for 10 minutes – this will keep it extra juicy and moist.

While the chicken is roasting, make the dressing. Put the egg yolk, garlic, anchovy fillets, mustard and water into a mixing bowl. Mix with a balloon whisk, making sure to break down any big lumps. Using a teaspoon, add a little of the oil. Whisk well to make sure it is fully incorporated, then repeat. This is quite painstaking, but it prevents the dressing splitting. If, at any point, the dressing starts to look overly shiny, add a few drops of lemon juice to loosen it, and continue adding the oil until it is all incorporated.

Add the natural yogurt, Parmesan and some fresh pepper. Add lemon juice to taste. (This will make more Caesar dressing than you need but it will keep in the fridge for three or four days.)

Put the romaine leaves into a large bowl. If you're feeding four, you'll need only two, but if it's six, you'll need three. Dollop over a few tablespoons of the dressing and toss the leaves with your fingers to coat them. Add the tomatoes and the avocado and gently mix together.

Tip on to a serving platter. Again with your fingers, start to pull the chicken (skin and all) into big chunks, and lay them on the leaves. Drizzle 2 tablespoons of the cooking juices over the salad and scatter with Parmesan shavings.

Lentil and Baked Goat's Cheese Salad with Tomato Dressing

SERVES 2

FOR THE LENTIL SALAD:

2 tablespoons extra virgin
olive oil

a knob of butter

1 small onion, finely chopped

1 rib of celery, finely chopped

1 green chilli, finely chopped

150g Puy lentils

2 bay leaves

10g fresh thyme

1 clove of garlic, finely grated

400ml cold water

sea salt and freshly ground
black pepper

2 firm goat's cheese rounds
(100g each)

FOR THE TOMATO DRESSING:

30g walnuts

3 ripe tomatoes

15ml red wine vinegar

1 clove of garlic, crushed

½ teaspoon ground cumin

½ teaspoon sweet smoked
paprika

80ml extra virgin olive oil

sea salt and freshly ground
black pepper

100g rocket leaves and a drizzle
of extra virgin olive oil,
to serve

Preheat the oven to 180°C/160°C fan.

Put 1 tablespoon of the oil and the butter into a medium-sized sauce-pan, over a medium heat. Add the onion, celery and green chilli and cook for 5 minutes. Rinse the lentils well under cold running water, and add to the saucepan. Add the bay leaves, thyme and garlic and stir together for a minute or two. Add the water to the pan and bring to a boil.

Turn down the heat and simmer the lentils for 20 to 25 minutes. Check they are al dente – if not, cook for another few minutes. If, at any point, the pan gets very low on water, add a little more; do not let it boil dry.

Remove from the heat, drain off any remaining water and remove the bay leaves and thyme stalks. Stir in the remaining tablespoon of oil, season with salt and pepper and set aside to cool.

While the lentils are cooking, line a baking sheet with non-stick baking paper and place the walnuts for the tomato dressing on one side. Pop into the oven for 10 minutes, then remove the tray, turn the walnuts and add the goat's cheese. After another 5 minutes or so, the walnuts should be perfectly toasted and the goat's cheese baking nicely. Remove the walnuts and put into a mini-chopper, return the goat's cheese to the oven and turn the heat down low.

Boil a kettle of water. Put the tomatoes into a mixing bowl just big enough to hold them snugly and pour the boiling water over them. Leave for 90 seconds, then pour the water away. Minding your fingers, peel the skin off the tomatoes, slice into quarters, scoop out the seeds and add the flesh to the mini-chopper with the walnuts. Add the red wine vinegar, garlic, cumin and paprika and blitz to a purée. Scoop out into a jug and whisk in the olive oil. Season to taste.

To serve, divide the rocket leaves between two plates. Top with the lentils, a round of goat's cheese and drizzle with the tomato dressing.

Grilled Halloumi and Kale Salad
with Tahini Yogurt Dressing

SERVES 2

FOR THE KALE SALAD:

100g kale leaves

½ teaspoon sea salt

30g blanched almonds

1 avocado, destoned and cut
into chunks

4 spring onions, thinly sliced

100g radishes, thinly sliced

seeds of 1 pomegranate

2 teaspoons sesame seeds

2 teaspoons black sesame seeds

FOR THE HALLOUMI:

1 teaspoon turmeric

1 teaspoon hot smoked paprika

3 tablespoons extra virgin olive oil

200g halloumi, cut into
1cm-thick slices

FOR THE TAHINI YOGURT
DRESSING:

25ml tahini

100ml Greek yogurt

½ a lemon, zest and juice

sea salt

2 tablespoons extra virgin
olive oil, to serve

Prep the kale by removing the stalks and any thick stems, and cut or tear into bite-size pieces. Put the leaves into a large mixing bowl and add the salt, crushing it between your fingers. With both hands, massage the leaves with the salt for a minute or two; it will suddenly feel much softer in your hands. Add all the other ingredients, mix together and set to one side.

Turn your grill to its hottest setting. Put the turmeric, paprika and oil into a bowl and mix. Add the halloumi and coat in the spices and oil.

Place the halloumi on a baking sheet and pop under the hot grill. Allow to cook for 3 to 4 minutes, then turn over and cook for another 3 to 4 minutes. Turn off the grill but leave the halloumi there to keep warm.

For the dressing, put all the ingredients into a bowl and mix with a whisk.

To serve, divide the salad between two bowls, add some dressing and top with the warm halloumi and an extra drizzle of oil.

Minestrone made with Bone Broth

This bone broth recipe takes 8.5 hours but it's simple to make and worth the wait for the flavour it gives the soup. The broth can also be made in advance and frozen.

SERVES 2

FOR THE BONE BROTH:

(This will make 2 to 2.5l of broth, enough for about 6 portions, so freeze the extra and defrost as required)

2kg beef bones

1 tablespoon tomato purée

2 medium onions, peeled and halved

1 tablespoon black peppercorns

5 cloves of garlic, peeled

1 bunch of fresh flat-leaf parsley

1 bunch of fresh thyme

30g dried mushrooms

FOR THE MINESTRONE:

2 tablespoons extra virgin olive oil

50g smoked pancetta, cubed

1 large onion, diced

2 ribs of celery, diced

3 cloves of garlic, sliced

1 large courgette, diced

½ a Savoy cabbage, shredded

5 large cavolo nero leaves, thinly sliced

1 x 200g tin of cannellini beans, drained and rinsed

1 x 200g tin of borlotti beans, drained and rinsed

5g chopped fresh basil

800ml beef bone broth

extra virgin olive oil, Parmesan cheese, basil leaves and freshly ground black pepper, to serve

Preheat the oven to 200°C/180°C fan.

Place the bones in a large roasting tin. Rub the tomato purée all over the bones and cook in the oven for 30 minutes, turning halfway through.

Transfer the roasted bones to a large stockpot, and add the onions, peppercorns, garlic, herbs and dried mushrooms. Pour cold water into the pot, making sure to cover all the bones. Put on the hob and bring the water just up to boiling point, but don't let it boil. Reduce the heat and keep at a very gentle simmer.

Every 20 minutes or so for the first two hours, use a large spoon to skim off any scum that forms. Every other time, add a splash of very cold water to the pot. This will shock the broth and any fat should rise to the surface, making it easier to skim off.

After this, you can reduce how often you check, but do keep half an eye on the stock, skimming as required and topping up if necessary. Leave to simmer for another 6 hours.

Remove the bones and sieve the broth through a piece of muslin or a fine sieve. Clean the stockpot and return the broth to it. Bring to the boil over a high heat to reduce the stock to about 2.5 litres. Keep 800ml for the recipe and freeze the rest in two batches.

Put the oil into a heavy-based saucepan and place over a medium heat. Add the pancetta, onion and celery. Cook slowly for about 10 minutes, gently stirring throughout, to allow the fat to render from the pancetta and the vegetables to soften and sweeten without taking on any colour, then add the garlic and cook for another 90 seconds.

Add the courgette, cabbage, cavolo nero, the cannellini and borlotti beans and basil and mix well. Cook for a couple of minutes, then add the bone broth and simmer for about 8 minutes.

To serve, divide between two big bowls, drizzle with a glug of olive oil, grate over some Parmesan, scatter with a few basil leaves and finish off with a twist of pepper (the soup should be salty enough with the pancetta and the Parmesan).

Chilled Cucumber and Avocado Soup

SERVES 2

1 cucumber, peeled and sliced (reserve 6 slices for decoration)

2 avocados, peeled and destoned

2 jalapeño peppers, halved and deseeded

4 spring onions, roughly chopped

20ml extra virgin olive oil

100g natural yogurt

40g crème fraîche

120ml chicken or vegetable broth

5–10g fresh dill

1 lemon, juice only

sea salt and freshly ground black pepper

extra virgin olive oil, dill sprigs, 1 tomato, deseeded and diced, and hot sauce, such as Cholula, to serve

Put all the ingredients for the soup into a food processor or blender and blitz for about 5 minutes until silky smooth. Scrape down any soup from the sides and blitz for another minute or two. Taste, and add a pinch of salt and some pepper, if you think it needs it.

To serve, divide between two bowls and top with a good drizzle of olive oil, the reserved cucumber slices, dill sprigs, tomato and a few dashes of hot sauce.

Prosciutto, Burrata and Tomato Salad with Basil Dressing

SERVES 2

80g prosciutto

1 burrata cheese (or buffalo mozzarella)

150g sun-blushed tomatoes (or cherry tomatoes, halved)

sea salt and freshly ground black pepper

a handful of basil leaves

FOR THE DRESSING:

60ml extra virgin olive oil

2 tablespoons balsamic vinegar

5g chopped fresh basil leaves

1 small clove of garlic, crushed to a paste

sea salt and freshly ground black pepper

small basil leaves, to serve

Place all the ingredients for the dressing in the small bowl of a food processor and whizz together until the basil is totally broken down in the oil. (You can keep any unused dressing in a sterilized jam jar and it will keep for five days in the fridge.)

To serve, lay out the prosciutto on a large platter, in folds and waves so that it can catch the dressing. Add the burrata and gently press down on it so that it bursts its skin. Put the tomatoes around the meat, season, and add the dressing and the small basil leaves before serving.

Smoked Mackerel Pâté, Bagna Cauda and Crudités

SERVES 2

FOR THE SMOKED MACKEREL PÂTÉ:

100g smoked mackerel

40g crème fraîche

½ teaspoon wholegrain mustard

½ a lemon, zest and juice

5g lemon thyme, leaves only

5g finely chopped fresh flat-leaf parsley

30ml double cream

sea salt and freshly ground black pepper

FOR THE BAGNA CAUDA:

4 cloves of garlic, thinly sliced

8–10 anchovies (approximately 1 small tin)

60ml extra virgin olive oil

80g butter, cold and cubed

1 tablespoon apple cider vinegar

1 teaspoon lemon juice

sea salt and freshly ground black pepper

CRUDITÉ OPTIONS:

cauliflower florets

asparagus spears

mangetouts

sugar snap peas

romaine lettuce hearts

celery sticks

cucumber sticks

radishes

chicory leaves

cherry tomatoes

To make the smoked mackerel pâté, put the mackerel, crème fraîche, mustard and lemon zest into the small bowl of a food processor and blitz until smooth. Add the herbs, the double cream, 1 tablespoon of lemon juice and some salt and pepper. If you like it with more of a tang, add more lemon juice. Remove from the food processor and set to one side.

To make the bagna cauda, put the garlic, anchovies and oil into a small saucepan and place over a low heat. Stir with a small whisk to stop anything burning and to help break down the anchovies. Once they have dissolved into the oil (after around 5 minutes), remove the pan from the heat and transfer the contents to the small bowl of the food processor. While it is running, drop in the cubes of cold butter one by one until you end up with a creamy sauce. Add the apple cider vinegar, the lemon juice and some salt and pepper and mix together.

The crudités can be anything you have in the fridge from the list opposite. Something really crunchy to contrast with the soft pâté and the bagna cauda dip is best.

Monkfish Skewers with Basil Pesto

SERVES 2

FOR THE MONKFISH SKEWERS:

300g monkfish, cut into 3cm-square chunks (cod or halibut would work well too)

1 yellow pepper, cut into 3cm chunks

1 courgette, cut into 3cm chunks

1 small aubergine, cut into 3cm chunks

1 red onion, cut into quarters, layers separated

3 tablespoons extra virgin olive oil

sea salt and freshly ground black pepper

FOR THE BASIL PESTO:

1 clove of garlic, chopped

25g roughly chopped fresh basil

50g pine nuts, toasted

100ml extra virgin olive oil

75g Parmesan cheese, grated

lemon wedges, to serve

You will need: 4 bamboo or metal skewers (soak bamboo skewers in cold water for half an hour to prevent them charring), and a large pestle and mortar (optional)

Put all the ingredients for the monkfish skewers into a large mixing bowl and mix gently, making sure that everything is covered in the oil, salt and pepper. On each skewer, alternate the fish and the vegetables, cover and place in the fridge.

Make the pesto. This is a classic for a reason, and is packed full of things that are really good for you. If you want to do it the traditional way, you will need a large pestle and mortar. Crush the garlic (a little pinch of salt may help you to get it going), then add the basil leaves and pine nuts little by little until you have a thick paste. Add the olive oil and part stir, part crush everything together. Add the Parmesan and mix well. Alternatively, put the garlic, basil and pine nuts into a food processor and blitz while slowly adding the oil, then transfer to a bowl and stir in the Parmesan. (If you have any left over, it can be kept in the fridge in an airtight container, under a layer of extra virgin olive oil, for a week.)

Heat a griddle pan until you can feel the heat coming off it when you hold your hand above it. Place the skewers on the pan and cook for 2 minutes, then rotate. Repeat twice until the skewers are cooked evenly.

To serve, divide between two plates, cover with the pesto and enjoy. A green leaf salad is ideal with this.

Courgetti Vongole

SERVES 2

FOR THE CLAMS:

600g clams

2 tablespoons extra virgin olive oil

10g butter

1 onion, finely diced

1 red chilli, finely chopped

3 cloves of garlic, finely chopped

½ teaspoon paprika

½ teaspoon dried basil

½ teaspoon dried oregano

1 tablespoon tomato purée

70g n'duja

1 x 400g tin of plum tomatoes

100g cherry tomatoes

10g roughly chopped fresh flat-leaf parsley

sea salt and freshly ground black pepper

FOR THE COURGETTI:

1 tablespoon extra virgin olive oil, plus extra for dizzling

2 large courgettes, spiralized

1 teaspoon dried oregano

You will need: a spiralizer

Check the clams and discard any with damaged shells and any that don't close when they are gently tapped. Rinse well to make sure they're clean.

Put the oil and butter for the clams into a large saucepan (with a lid) and place on a low heat. Add the onion and chilli and cook gently for 10 minutes, until the onion has softened. Add the garlic and cook for another 90 seconds, then add the dried herbs and the tomato purée and cook for another 2 minutes.

Add the n'duja and stir to help it break up a little. Once it has dissolved down to a thick sauce, add the tinned and cherry tomatoes and turn up the heat. Just as the tomato sauce starts to boil, add the clams and put the lid on quickly. Give the pan a gentle shake to make sure all the clams get some heat. After 3 minutes, take the lid off – the shells should all have burst open. Discard any that remain closed. Turn the heat right down to a simmer while you cook the courgetti.

Put the oil in a wok, or heavy-based frying pan, heat, and add the spiralized courgettes and oregano, tossing them quickly for about 3 minutes. You want them to be starting to soften but to retain their crunch.

Tip the courgetti noodles into the clam pot and cover with the tomato sauce. Add the parsley and season to taste.

Before serving, toss the clams, courgetti and sauce one last time and divide between two big pasta bowls. Drizzle with a little extra virgin olive oil, then serve.

Karahi Prawns

SERVES 2

1 tablespoon ghee

3 tablespoons extra virgin olive oil

1 onion, finely chopped

2 cloves of garlic, finely chopped

5cm piece of ginger, finely chopped

2 green chillies, finely chopped

4 large, ripe tomatoes, chopped

350g king prawns, shelled (fresh or defrosted from frozen)

1½ tablespoons garam masala

1 lemon, juice only

sea salt and freshly ground black pepper

2 tablespoons natural yogurt, to serve

Put the ghee and oil into a frying pan and cook over a medium heat. Once hot, add the onion and cook for 5 to 10 minutes until it has softened and is starting to go golden brown. Add the garlic and stir for 30 seconds.

Add the ginger, chillies and tomatoes and cook for around 10 minutes, stirring regularly to make sure nothing catches or burns. If it starts to look a little dry, add a splash of water. The tomatoes will begin to form a sauce.

Add the prawns and garam masala and mix well. Cook for 5 minutes, stirring and flipping the prawns to make sure they cook on both sides. Turn off the heat and squeeze in the lemon juice. Check the seasoning and add salt and pepper, if needed.

To serve, divide between two plates and add a spoonful of natural yogurt to each one.

This is delicious with vegetable rice (see p.330) and a Punjabi salad (see p.332).

Mediterranean Fish with Vegetable Hash and Aioli

SERVES 2

FOR THE FISH GRILL:

8 anchovies (approximately 1 small tin)

2 tablespoons capers

6 tablespoons extra virgin olive oil

4 cloves of garlic, finely grated

4 red chillies, finely chopped

sea salt and freshly ground black pepper

200g salmon fillet

200g seabass fillet

4 king prawns

2 lemons, juice only

FOR THE VEGETABLE HASH:

3 tablespoons extra virgin olive oil

20g butter

½ a cauliflower, chopped into small chunks

1 medium sweet potato, grated

50g green beans, topped and tailed and chopped

1 green chilli, finely chopped

1 tablespoon dried oregano

3 cloves of garlic, finely grated

sea salt and freshly ground black pepper

FOR THE AIOLI:

1 large egg yolk

1 small clove of garlic, crushed to a paste

1 teaspoon Dijon mustard

1 teaspoon cold water

175ml extra virgin olive oil

½ a lemon, juice only

sea salt and freshly ground black pepper

Preheat the oven to 160°C/140°C fan.

Put the anchovies, capers and 5 tablespoons of the oil into a small saucepan and place on a gentle heat to warm through, stirring occasionally to break down the anchovies. Cook for about 10 minutes, then add the garlic and red chillies, salt and pepper. Turn off the heat and leave to one side for the flavours to infuse.

You can make the aioli in advance, as this will keep in a sterilized airtight jar or tub for up to two weeks. Put the egg yolk, garlic, mustard and water into a medium-sized mixing bowl and whisk together. Using a teaspoon, add a little of the oil. Whisk well to make sure it is fully incorporated, then repeat. This is quite painstaking, but it prevents the dressing splitting. If, at any point, the dressing starts to look overly shiny, add a few drops of lemon juice to loosen it, and continue with the oil until it is all incorporated. Taste and add lemon juice and salt and pepper, as needed.

To make the vegetable hash, put the oil and butter into a large pan and place over a medium heat. Add the cauliflower, sweet potato and beans and cook for 7 to 8 minutes, stirring frequently. Add the green chilli, oregano and garlic, salt and pepper, and cook for another 5 minutes.

Heat a griddle pan until it is smoking hot. While it's heating, put the salmon, seabass and prawns into a mixing bowl and coat with 1 tablespoon of the oil and a little salt and pepper. Place the salmon and the seabass on to the hot griddle skin side down, and cook for 2 minutes, then flip the seabass and cook the other side for 1 minute and remove to a warm serving plate. Add the prawns in its place. Once the salmon has had about 5 minutes on its first side, flip that over, cook for a further 2 minutes and then remove to join the seabass. The prawns will need 2 to 3 minutes on each side, depending on their size. Make sure they are evenly cooked and are pink all over before removing them from the pan.

Pour the garlic and anchovy dressing over the fish.

Serve with the hash and a good dollop of aioli. This would also be great with some steamed broccoli or leafy greens.

Whole Roast Salmon with Lemon Herby Stuffing

SERVES 10

2 tablespoons extra virgin olive oil

1 whole salmon, approximately 2kg, gutted

150g butter, softened

2 banana shallots, finely diced

3 cloves of garlic, grated

2 lemons, zest and juice

10g finely chopped fresh tarragon leaves

10g finely chopped fresh flat-leaf parsley

sea salt and freshly ground black pepper

5 bay leaves

Preheat the oven to 160°C/140°C fan.

Line a large roasting tin with non-stick baking paper. Rub the oil all over the outside of the salmon and lay it in the tin.

Put the softened butter into a large mixing bowl and, with a wooden spoon, beat in all the other ingredients, apart from the bay leaves. With your hands, shape the stuffing into a rough sausage shape the length of the cavity in the salmon, lay the bay leaves evenly on top of the stuffing, and place it inside, down the length of the fish.

Cut 5 pieces of butcher's string, long enough to go around the fish, and tie around the salmon at intervals to keep the belly sealed. Wrap a little tin foil over the tail to stop it burning.

Place the salmon in the oven and cook for half an hour, then take out and spoon over all the lovely buttery, herby juices. Turn the oven up to 210°C/190°C fan and return the salmon to the oven for a final 8 minutes.

When it is cooked, carefully remove the string and gently lift the salmon out of the tin and place on a large serving dish. Spoon over some of the juices and serve immediately.

This would be perfect with a green salad or roast vegetables – whatever you fancy.

Cauliflower Steaks with Feta

SERVES 2

1 large cauliflower
2 tablespoons extra virgin olive oil
2 teaspoons za'atar
sea salt and freshly ground black pepper

150g feta cheese, crumbled, 2 teaspoons chipotle chilli flakes, 2 tablespoons extra virgin olive oil and 1 tablespoon fresh oregano leaves, to serve

Preheat the oven to 200°C/180°C fan.

Line a baking sheet with non-stick baking paper.

Take the cauliflower and turn it stalk up on a chopping board. You want to get two cauliflower steaks, each about 2 centimetres thick, with the stalk holding them together, so slice off the side florets and save those for another day, to make cauliflower rice or eat as crudités, for example.

Put the two steaks side by side on the baking paper and drizzle with the oil and za'atar. Rub with your hands to make sure both sides are evenly covered and add a little salt and pepper.

Cook in the oven for 20 to 25 minutes. The steaks should be golden brown and starting to char around the edges.

To serve, cover each steak with feta, sprinkle with chilli flakes, drizzle with olive oil and scatter with the oregano.

Cauliflower Cheese with Crispy Shallots

SERVES 2

FOR THE CAULIFLOWER CHEESE:

½ a cauliflower, broken into florets

½ a Romanesco cauliflower, broken into florets

3 tablespoons extra virgin olive oil

20g butter, plus extra for greasing

1 large leek, thinly sliced

2 cloves of garlic, finely grated

400ml double cream

1 tablespoon Dijon mustard

½ a nutmeg, grated

120g mature Cheddar cheese, grated

30g Parmesan cheese, grated

30g ground almonds

sea salt and freshly ground black pepper

FOR THE CRISPY SHALLOTS:

2 tablespoons ghee

2 tablespoons extra virgin olive oil

4 banana shallots, very finely sliced

Preheat the oven to 190°C/170°C fan.

Bring a large saucepan of salted water to the boil. Add both cauliflowers and cook for 5 minutes. Drain and leave to steam dry in a colander.

Rinse the saucepan, put the oil, butter and the sliced leek into it and place over a medium heat. Cook for 8 to 10 minutes until the leek starts to soften and lose some of its water content – you don't want a watery cauliflower cheese!

Add the garlic and stir for 90 seconds, then add the cream, mustard and nutmeg and cook until the cream has reduced by a third. Add the cauliflower and half the grated Cheddar and mix well. Remove from the heat.

Butter a 26cm-long, deep pie dish, pour in the cauliflower mix and sprinkle with the rest of the Cheddar.

Put the Parmesan, ground almonds and some salt and pepper into a small dish, mix together and pour over the cauliflower. Place the dish on a baking sheet in case it spills over, and cook in the oven for 25 to 30 minutes, until golden and bubbling.

While this is baking, put the ghee and the oil for the crispy shallots into a frying pan and melt over a medium heat. Add the shallots and fry for 25 to 30 minutes, stirring occasionally; the shallots at the edges of the pan will brown more quickly. When they are all a deep golden brown, lift them out with a slotted spoon and drain on kitchen paper to crisp up.

Sprinkle the cauliflower cheese with the crispy shallots.

Serve in all its cheesy, crispy glory with a peppery green salad – try mixing spinach, watercress and chicory leaves.

Slow-cooked Black Dal with Homemade Paneer and Charred Broccoli

This isn't a quick recipe (12 hours soaking, and 13 hours cooking) but it's mostly hands-off time and the end result is delicious. This is a great one to make a lot of, and somehow it tastes even better on the second day. Any extra can also be frozen.

SERVES 10

FOR THE BLACK DAL:

600g urad dal (or black lentils)

50g butter

4 tablespoons extra virgin olive oil

2 onions, finely chopped

1 head of garlic, cloves peeled and grated

5cm piece of ginger, finely grated

2 tablespoons tomato purée

2 teaspoons cumin seeds, toasted and ground

2 teaspoons coriander seeds, toasted and ground

1 teaspoon black peppercorns, toasted and ground

½ teaspoon cayenne pepper

½ teaspoon turmeric

2 bay leaves

1 cinnamon stick

2 x 400g tin of plum tomatoes

400ml single cream

100ml double cream

sea salt and freshly ground black pepper

FOR THE PANEER:

1.5 litres whole milk

1 lemon, juice only

1 tablespoon ghee

½ teaspoon turmeric

FOR THE BROCCOLI:

200g tenderstem or purple sprouting broccoli

1 tablespoon extra virgin olive oil

You will need: 2 pieces of muslin

Soak the dal according to the packet instructions – usually, the day before, in plenty of cold water, for a minimum of 12 hours.

Preheat the oven to 140°C/120°C fan.

Rinse the dal, place in a large saucepan and cover with cold water. Bring to the boil and simmer gently for an hour. A little foam or scum may form on the surface: skim it off with a large metal spoon and discard.

While the dal is cooking, put the butter and oil into a large casserole pot (with a lid that can go into the oven) over a gentle heat. Add the onions and cook for 10 minutes, until they have softened. Add the garlic, stir for a couple of minutes, then add the ginger and the tomato purée. Cook for another 2 minutes and, when the purée has darkened, add all the spices. Mix well, then add the tomatoes. As they start to cook, press them against the side of the casserole pot with the back of a wooden spoon to burst them. Continue cooking very gently until the dal is cooked (1 hour).

Drain the dal and add to the casserole pot. Combine well. Add the single cream, 200ml of water and a little salt and pepper – once the dal has had its full cooking time, you can balance the seasoning.

Transfer the casserole pot, with its lid on, to the oven and cook for 6 hours, then remove the lid and cook for another 6 hours. Stir occasionally. If it starts to get a little dry, add a splash more water, but not too much – you want thick, dark, delicious dal.

Meanwhile, double-line a colander with muslin and put it into the sink. Heat the milk for the panner in a saucepan and, when it starts steaming, add the lemon juice and stir. It should curdle almost immediately. Pour the curds and whey gently into the colander, then pour over a jug of cold water to rinse the curds.

Gather up the corners of the muslin, twisting them until you end up with a tight ball, and squeeze out as much liquid as you can. Place the paneer into a plastic pot, level it out, then place another empty pot on top and weight it with two tins. Place it in the fridge for 2 hours until set.

An hour before you are ready to serve, take the dal out of the oven and add the double cream for that next level of richness. Return to the oven and increase the heat to 160°C/140°C fan.

When you are ready to eat, remove the paneer from the fridge, tip it out on to a cutting board and cut into chunky cubes. Place the ghee in a frying pan on a gentle heat, then add the turmeric. Add the cubes of paneer and fry each side for a minute. They should take on a lovely yellow from the turmeric and a golden edge from the heat.

Rub the broccoli with the oil, heat a griddle pan and place the broccoli on it, pressing down with the back of a spatula to make sure it's in contact with the pan. Turn after a few minutes and repeat.

To serve, ladle out some of the dal into big bowls, and top with the fried paneer and the griddled broccoli.

Dad's Dal

SERVES 2

150g split red lentils

1 tablespoon ghee

2 tablespoons extra virgin olive oil

1 onion, chopped

5cm piece of ginger, finely chopped

2 cloves of garlic, finely chopped

1 green chilli, chopped

3 tomatoes, chopped

2 teaspoons ground coriander

1 teaspoon garam masala

1 teaspoon ground ginger

2 cloves

1 teaspoon freshly ground black pepper

1 lemon, juice only

sea salt to taste

natural yogurt and coriander leaves, to serve

Put the lentils into a medium-sized saucepan and cover with cold water. Bring the water up to the boil, then simmer for approximately 15 minutes until al dente.

While the lentils are simmering, put the ghee and the oil into a frying pan over a low heat. Add the onion and ginger and fry until the onion starts to turn golden brown. After about 10 minutes, add the garlic and chilli, then the tomatoes and spices. Stir well and cook for a further 5 to 10 minutes until the tomatoes have cooked down and softened into a sauce.

By now, the lentils should be done. Drain in a colander and add to the tomatoes. Stir together and cook for another 2 to 3 minutes.

Squeeze over the lemon juice, and add salt, to taste.

To serve, divide between two bowls and add some yogurt.

Delicious on its own, but if you want to turn it into something more substantial, it also goes well with vegetable rice (see p.330) and a Punjabi salad (see p.332).

Dinners

Cheese Burgers

SERVES 2

320g steak, minced – for maximum flavour, try a combination of ribeye and short rib

sea salt and freshly ground black pepper

20g butter

2 tablespoons extra virgin olive oil

1 red onion, thinly sliced

4 slices of cheese – try mature Cheddar, Brie or Camembert

1 beef tomato, sliced

1 avocado, destoned and sliced

OTHER OPTIONS:

100g spinach, wilted

hot sauce

crispy bacon

jalapeños

fried egg

lettuce

quick pickles (see page 335)

You can either buy the steak and mince it yourself, or ask your butcher to do it for you. You want a good mix of meat and fat to get maximum flavour. Add salt and pepper and shape into two burgers. Allow to rest and come up to room temperature.

Put the butter and oil into a frying pan on a medium heat. When the butter has melted, add the red onion. Stir to break it up, then cook for 20 minutes, stirring every 5 minutes, so the onion becomes soft and caramelized.

When the onion is ready, heat a skillet and, when it's hot, place the burgers on it. You don't need to oil the pan; there should be enough fat in the burgers. For medium rare, cook for 3 minutes each side on a high heat. For a well-done burger, cook for 6 to 7 minutes each side. When you flip the burger, place the cheese on top so it starts to melt from the heat of the burger.

Top each burger topped with a slice of beef tomato, slices of avocado and some caramelized onions, or choose from the list of options. Serve with a green salad.

Steak with Béarnaise Sauce and Griddled Broccoli

SERVES 2

FOR THE STEAK:

sea salt and freshly ground
black pepper

360g bavette steak, as one piece

30g butter

2 tablespoons extra virgin
olive oil

3 tablespoons white wine vinegar

5 black peppercorns

2 egg yolks

½ a lemon, juice only

2 tablespoons chopped fresh
tarragon

sea salt

FOR THE BÉARNAISE SAUCE:

150g butter

1 banana shallot, very finely
chopped

FOR THE GRIDDLED BROCCOLI:

1 tablespoon extra virgin olive oil

120g tenderstem broccoli

First of all, clarify the butter for the Béarnaise sauce, by melting it slowly in a small saucepan over a low heat. The milk solids will settle at the bottom and you can pour off the clarified butter with ease.

Put the shallot, vinegar and black peppercorns into another small pan and place on the heat. Watching it all the time, reduce the vinegar to about 3 teaspoons, then sieve.

Once it is cool, add 2 teaspoons of the vinegar reduction to the egg yolks, along with a teaspoon of water and a few drops of lemon juice. Use a balloon whisk to bring it all together. This should only take a few seconds.

Place this bowl over a bain-marie (a pan of water at simmering point; the bowl should fit into but not touch the water). Don't let the water get too hot; you don't want to scramble the egg. Slowly add the clarified butter to the yolks, whisking continuously, as you would when making mayonnaise. Each addition should be incorporated before the next is added. If it starts looking overly shiny, or looks as if it may be cooking, add a few drops of lemon juice or a few drops of cold water.

When the sauce is lovely and thick, remove from the heat and add the tarragon. Taste and season with a little salt, if needed. Keep to one side, stirring occasionally to stop a skin forming.

Season both sides of the steak. Put the butter and oil into a frying pan and place on a medium heat. Once the butter is foaming, add the steak. Use a spoon to pour the hot butter over the top of the steak as it cooks. After 3 minutes, turn the steak and repeat, then remove to a chopping board to rest.

Wipe the frying pan and return to the heat. Rub the oil over the broccoli and put into the pan. To get maximum contact, press or weight the broccoli down, using the back of a turner or even another pan. After 2 minutes turn the broccoli over and cook on the other side. Repeat until it's started to soften and char all over, then remove to a platter.

The steak should now be ready to slice. Carve it into half-centimetre-thick slices and put on the platter with the broccoli.

Spoon on the Béarnaise sauce and serve immediately.

Meatballs in a Roast Tomato and Garlic Sauce with Sweet Potato Noodles

SERVES 2

FOR THE MEATBALLS:

200g beef mince

200g pork mince

1 tablespoon dried oregano

1 tablespoon chopped fresh basil

sea salt and freshly ground black pepper

10g butter

3 tablespoons extra virgin olive oil

FOR THE TOMATO AND GARLIC SAUCE:

8 ripe tomatoes, on the vine

2 strands of cherry tomatoes, on the vine

1 red onion, sliced into 6 wedges

1 head of garlic, broken into cloves

4 sprigs of rosemary

3 tablespoons extra virgin olive oil

100ml red wine

2 tablespoons balsamic vinegar

1 tablespoon chopped fresh basil

FOR THE NOODLES:

2–3 sweet potatoes, spiralized

2 tablespoons extra virgin olive oil

You will need: a spiralizer

Preheat the oven to 200°C/180°C fan.

Place all the ingredients for the meatballs, except the butter and oil, into a mixing bowl and, with your hands, mix and knead together. Shape the mince into just bigger than golfball-sized balls – you should make around 12. Cover and place in the fridge.

Line a roasting tin with baking paper and put into it all the tomatoes, the onion, garlic and rosemary. Coat everything with the oil and season well. Place in the hot oven and roast for 25 minutes. Remove the tin, give everything a quick stir, then roast for another 20 minutes. The tomatoes should have burst their skins and the juices will have collected in the pan. Place the tomatoes and their juices into a large saucepan (removing the vines), along with the onion and the soft flesh of the garlic (squeezed from its skins). Using a stick blender, blend everything together to make a smooth sauce.

Heat gently, add the red wine and balsamic vinegar and simmer for 20 minutes.

After 10 minutes, put the butter and oil for the meatballs into a large frying pan and place on the heat. Add the meatballs and cook for 6 to 8 minutes, turning them and shaking the pan so they cook evenly. Turn off the heat.

Add the basil to the tomato sauce and stir through. Add the meatballs and turn them over in the sauce to coat well. Return the pan to a gentle heat to keep warm.

Place the meatball pan back on the heat; it should have some lovely cooking juices in it. Add the sweet potato noodles and the oil and turn up the heat. You want to cook the sweet potato noodles quite quickly so they don't go soggy. Toss and flip them in the pan for 5 to 7 minutes.

To serve, divide the noodles between two bowls and top with the meatballs and the sauce.

Cottage Pie with Cauliflower Mash

SERVES 2

FOR THE COTTAGE PIE:

3 tablespoons extra virgin olive oil

a knob of butter

1 large onion, finely chopped

2 ribs of celery, chopped

3 cloves of garlic, finely grated

1 teaspoon dried basil

1 tablespoon tomato purée

400g beef mince

300ml beef stock

3 sprigs of thyme

3 bay leaves

sea salt and freshly ground black pepper

FOR THE CAULIFLOWER MASH:

1 large cauliflower, broken into florets

40g crème fraîche

60g butter, cold and cubed

¼ of a nutmeg, grated

sea salt and freshly ground black pepper

Preheat the oven to 190°C/170°C fan.

Heat the oil and butter for the cottage pie in a saucepan, then add the onion and celery and cook for 5 minutes to soften. Add the garlic, basil and tomato purée and cook for 90 seconds or so. Add the mince and mix together well, breaking down any lumps with the back of a wooden spoon.

Next, add the beef stock and the herbs. Bring up to the boil, then reduce the heat and simmer for 20 minutes.

While that is cooking, steam the cauliflower for 6 minutes, then allow to steam dry in a colander. After a few minutes put the florets into a large saucepan and, using a potato masher, crush them, but leaving some texture. Add the crème fraîche, butter and nutmeg and mix well.

Place the pan on a low heat for 5 minutes so that any excess water evaporates, stirring regularly. Season with salt and pepper.

When the mince is ready, remove the bay leaves and thyme stalks. Use a slotted spoon to transfer the mince into an ovenproof pie dish and level it out. Spoon over a few tablespoons of the gravy. (Save the rest for serving.) Cover the mince with the cauliflower mash and cook in the oven for 25 minutes, until golden brown and bubbling.

Serve with green vegetables and more gravy.

Harissa Lamb Chops

SERVES 2

FOR THE HARISSA:

(This will make double what you need, but it will keep in the fridge for a week. It's also delicious rubbed over a chicken and roasted)

4 tablespoons extra virgin olive oil

4 cloves of garlic, finely grated

2 red chillies, finely chopped

4 tablespoons dried red pepper flakes

2 teaspoons ground cumin

1 teaspoon ground coriander

60g tomato purée

1 red pepper, roasted

1 teaspoon sweet smoked paprika

15g chopped fresh coriander

1 teaspoon chipotle chilli flakes (optional)

FOR THE CHOPS:

4 lamb chops, thick cut

Put the oil into a small saucepan and place over a low heat. Add the garlic, chillies and pepper flakes and allow to warm through and infuse the oil, for around 5 minutes.

After 5 minutes, add the spices and tomato purée. Mix and continue to heat gently for a few minutes.

Remove the pan from the heat and add the red pepper, paprika and fresh coriander. Using a stick blender, blitz everything together into a thick paste. If you like more heat and a smoky taste, add the chipotle flakes.

Rub half the harissa over the lamb chops and marinate for a minimum of 4 hours.

To cook the chops, heat a frying pan over a medium heat. Stand the lamb chops up, side by side, fat down, in the pan. The fat will start to render and provide enough oil to cook the chops. Leave them for 4 to 5 minutes. Lay the chops down on one side and cook for 2 to 5 minutes (depending on how well you like them done), then flip and cook the other side for another 2 to 5 minutes.

Allow to rest for 5 minutes before serving, with cabbage thoran (see p.336) or some tray-baked roast vegetables (see p.334).

Karahi Lamb

SERVES 2

1 tablespoon ghee

3 tablespoons extra virgin olive oil

300g lamb leg, cut into 2.5cm chunks

sea salt and freshly ground black pepper

1 onion, finely chopped

4 cloves of garlic, finely chopped

5cm piece of ginger, finely chopped

2 green chillies, finely chopped

5 large ripe tomatoes, chopped

1 tablespoon garam masala

1 teaspoon freshly ground coriander

1 teaspoon freshly ground black pepper

1 tablespoon balsamic vinegar

Put the ghee and oil into a frying pan and place over a medium heat. Season the lamb with salt and pepper and, when the pan is hot, add to the ghee and oil. Brown the meat on all sides, then transfer to a plate.

Put the onion into the frying pan. Cook for 5 to 8 minutes until it has softened and started to go golden brown. Add the garlic and stir for 30 seconds.

Add the ginger, chillies and tomatoes. Cook for 2 minutes, then return the lamb to the pan. Coat it in the sauce, then cover the pan with a lid and simmer for 15 minutes. The tomatoes will break down and create a sauce. Check occasionally; you may need to add a little water to stop it becoming too thick and dry.

Add the spices and pepper and cook for another 5 minutes. Turn off the heat and add the balsamic vinegar. Check the seasoning and add a little salt, to taste.

To serve, divide between two bowls and serve with vegetable rice (see p.330) and a Punjabi salad (see p.332).

Lamb Stew

SERVES 4

2 tablespoons extra virgin olive oil

a knob of butter

800g lamb neck, bone in

1 red onion, diced

2 ribs of celery, finely diced

3 cloves of garlic, finely grated

12 shallots, peeled and left whole

150ml red wine

500ml lamb or beef stock

5 sprigs of thyme

10g chopped fresh flat-leaf parsley

2 bay leaves

150g button mushrooms

sea salt and freshly ground black pepper

Preheat the oven to 170°C/150°C fan.

Put the oil and butter into a casserole pot and place on the heat. Brown the lamb neck on all sides. Remove from the pan and add the red onion and celery. Cook for 5 minutes until they begin to soften, then add the garlic and shallots and mix well.

Turn up the heat and add the red wine to the pan. Scrape up any bits that have stuck to the bottom and reduce the wine until it just coats the onion. Put the lamb neck back into the pot and add the stock. It should cover the lamb; if it doesn't, top up with water. Add the herbs and place in the oven for an hour, with the lid on.

Remove the casserole pot from the oven and give everything a good stir. Add the button mushrooms and return to the oven for another 45 minutes to an hour, with the lid off. The meat should now be falling from the bone and be really soft and tender. Remove the meat and veg with a slotted spoon and keep to one side, then return the sauce to the pan. Place over a high heat and reduce until the volume is halved. Return the lamb and vegetables to the sauce and mix well.

Serve with a vegetable mash and buttery greens.

Pulled Pork and Crackling Lettuce Wraps

SERVES 8 TO 10

FOR THE PULLED PORK:

3 large onions, thickly sliced

1 head of garlic, broken into cloves

200ml vegetable stock

1 tablespoon chilli powder

1 teaspoon ground cumin

1 teaspoon ground cinnamon

2 tablespoons sea salt

3.5kg shoulder of pork, neck end, bone in and skin scored finely

1 tablespoon smoked paprika

3 tablespoons extra virgin olive oil

quick pickles (see page 335), fresh coriander leaves, 4 romaine lettuces, sliced in half and pulled into leaves, to serve

Preheat your oven to the highest setting, around 250°C/230°C fan.

Line the base of a large roasting tin with silver foil, then put in the sliced onions, garlic and the vegetable stock (this is just to keep the vegetables moist at the first stage of cooking).

Mix together the spices, apart from the paprika, and rub all over the flesh of the pork shoulder, avoiding the skin. Rub the salt into the scores on the skin and place the pork in the roasting tin on top of the onions and garlic.

Cook in the oven for 15 minutes, then turn the heat right down to 140°C/120°C fan and leave to cook for 1 hour. Rotate the tray and return to the oven for another hour. Repeat this for a total of 5 hours; by this point the flesh should be really juicy and tender and ready to be pulled. Remove the tray from the oven and turn it back up to 250°C/230°C fan. Once it's hot, return the pork for a final 15 minutes to re-crisp the crackling.

Remove the meat from the tin and put on to a large chopping board. Slice off the crackling and keep to one side (if it's not fully crackled, put it back in the oven on a high heat for 5 more minutes). With two forks, start pulling the meat off the bones, shredding it as you go. Stir through the smoked paprika and the olive oil and a spoonful of the cooking juices. Place the meat on a platter and chop up the crackling.

Serve with the pickles, coriander leaves and lettuce wraps.

Korean Stir-fried Pork Belly with Broccoli Kimchi Rice

SERVES 4

1kg pork belly, skin removed

2 tablespoons ghee

4 tablespoons extra virgin olive oil

1 onion, thinly sliced

10g butter

4 eggs

3 tablespoons sesame seeds

1 bunch of spring onions, thinly sliced

FOR THE MARINADE:

1 onion, sliced

5cm piece of ginger, peeled and chopped

3 cloves of garlic, sliced

2 tablespoons Korean chilli paste (gochujang)

2 tablespoons Korean soya bean paste (sunjang ssamjang)

2 tablespoons Korean chilli flakes (gochugaru)

2 tablespoons rice wine vinegar

2 tablespoons mirin

2 tablespoons fish sauce

FOR THE BROCCOLI KIMCHI RICE:

broccoli rice (see p.330)

100g quick kimchi (see p.327)

2 tablespoons extra virgin olive oil

Place the pork belly in the freezer for an hour; this will make it easier to slice.

Once the pork is semi-frozen, slice it as thinly as possible with a very sharp knife – ideally, only a millimetre or two thick – and place in a large mixing bowl.

Put all the ingredients for the marinade into a jug and use a stick blender to blitz together. Pour it over the sliced pork and massage it into the meat, making sure it's all covered. Cover the bowl and allow it to marinate in the fridge for 30 minutes.

Start to cook the broccoli rice about 15 minutes before you want to eat. Put the oil into a frying pan, add the broccoli rice and kimchi and mix well until hot. Continue cooking for another couple of minutes, then place in a serving bowl.

Heat a wok and put in the ghee and 2 tablespoons of oil. Add the strips of pork belly in batches and fry quickly. You don't want the pork to stew or dry out. Then add the onion. Fire up a small frying pan, and put in the butter and the remaining 2 tablespoons of oil to fry the eggs. Once hot, crack in the eggs and, when cooked, place on top of the broccoli kimchi rice.

Tip the pork into a serving bowl and scatter with the sesame seeds and spring onions.

Serve with the fried eggs and broccoli rice.

Pork Chops with Sage Butter

SERVES 2

2 pork chops, 3cm thick, skin removed

sea salt and freshly ground black pepper

50g butter

2 tablespoons extra virgin olive oil

12 sage leaves

Take each pork chop and score through the fat, nearly to the flesh, so that it will render more quickly and add to the cooking flavours. Season the chops with salt and pepper and put to one side.

Put the butter and oil into a frying pan and place on a medium heat. Once hot, add the chops and fry for 6 minutes. Turn the chops and add the sage leaves. The leaves may spit a little in the hot butter, but that will soon stop. Baste the chop with the butter and sage leaves and cook for another 6 minutes.

Turn the chops on to the side with the fat and hold them with some tongs for 4 to 5 minutes.

Remove from the heat and allow to rest for at least 5 minutes before serving.

To serve, drizzle over some sage butter and enjoy with some mixed green vegetables (see p.325) or a leek and courgette gratin (see p.335).

Tandoori Masala Salmon with Raita

SERVES 2

FOR THE TANDOORI SALMON:

3 tablespoons tandoori masala powder

300g salmon fillet

30g butter

2 tablespoons extra virgin olive oil

FOR THE RAITA:

½ a cucumber, diced

250g natural yogurt

5g chopped fresh mint leaves

½ a teaspoon dried mint

½ a lemon, juice only

sea salt and freshly ground black pepper

4 iceberg lettuce leaves, 1 onion, finely diced, 5g finely chopped fresh coriander, to serve

Rub the tandoori masala powder all over the flesh of the salmon, then set to one side.

To make the raita, put all the ingredients into a bowl and mix well.

Put the butter and oil into a frying pan and place over a medium heat. Once the butter starts foaming, put the salmon into the pan, skin side down. Cook for around 8 minutes. Baste the top of the fish with the butter and oil while it's cooking, then flip it over. Cook the fish flesh side down for another 90 seconds. Remove from the heat.

To serve, take the skin off the salmon. Take a lettuce leaf and load it with the salmon. Top with the raita, onion and coriander.

Spicy Salmon Curry

SERVES 2

FOR THE SALMON:
300g salmon fillet, skin removed
1 teaspoon turmeric
1 teaspoon sea salt
2 tablespoons extra virgin olive oil
1 teaspoon ghee

FOR THE SAUCE:
4 tablespoons extra virgin olive oil

1 tablespoon ghee
1 tablespoon black mustard seeds
3 cloves of garlic
1 green chilli, finely chopped
4 large tomatoes, finely chopped
1 teaspoon mustard powder
1 teaspoon chilli powder

Cut the salmon into big bite-size cubes and rub them with the turmeric and salt. (You may want to use gloves for this, as turmeric can stain your hands yellow.)

Put the oil and ghee for the salmon into a frying pan and place on a medium heat. Add the salmon and shallow fry for 1 minute on each side, then remove from the pan.

Put 2 tablespoons of the oil and the ghee for sauce into the pan, add the mustard seeds, garlic and chilli and cook over a medium to high heat. Fry for 30 seconds, stirring continuously – you don't want the mustard seeds or garlic to burn.

Add the tomatoes and stir on a high heat for a couple of minutes, then turn down to low. Stir occasionally. After 5 minutes, add the mustard and chilli powders and 100ml of water.

Stir for another 5 to 10 minutes. Return the salmon to the pan with any juices and the remaining oil to the pan and stir gently. Simmer for 2 minutes. Taste and season with salt, if needed.

Serve with cauliflower rice (see p.330), yogurt and a Punjabi salad (see p.332).

Thai-style Mussels and King Prawns

SERVES 2

400g mussels (fresh or defrosted from frozen)

200g king prawns, shelled (fresh or defrosted from frozen)

1 banana shallot

3 cloves of garlic

3cm piece of ginger

1 lemongrass stalk

1 red chilli

10g chopped fresh coriander

2 tablespoons coconut oil

400ml coconut milk

2 tablespoons fish sauce

1 tablespoon soy sauce

3 kaffir lime leaves

100g white cabbage, shredded

100g green beans, topped and tailed

50g cherry tomatoes, whole

100g beansprouts

a handful of chopped fresh Thai basil

40g unsalted peanuts, toasted and chopped, and Thai basil leaves, to serve

You will need: a wok or large pan with a lid

First, prep the seafood. Remove any beards and barnacles the mussels may have and check they are all alive – they should all be shut or close when gently tapped. De-vein the prawns by running a knife along their backs and removing the waste tube.

Place the banana shallot, garlic, ginger, lemongrass, chilli and coriander in a mini-chopper and blitz it into a paste.

Heat a wok or large pan with a lid, and add the coconut oil. Add the paste and cook for 2 minutes on a high heat. Stir for another minute to prevent anything burning. Add the coconut milk, fish and soy sauces and turn the heat down to a simmer. Add the kaffir lime leaves.

Simmer for 15 minutes, or until it has reduced by a third.

Turn the heat back up and, when at boiling point, add the mussels and prawns. Pop the lid on and give the pan a gentle shake. Cook on high for 3 minutes, by which point the mussels should all have opened. If any mussels remain closed after cooking, discard.

Add the vegetables and the chopped Thai basil and cook for another 3 minutes.

To serve, divide between two bowls, and sprinkle with some peanuts and Thai basil leaves.

Pan-fried Cod with Clams

SERVES 2

FOR THE COD:

20g butter

1 tablespoon extra virgin olive oil

2 cod fillets, skin on, each weighing about 160g

sea salt and freshly ground black pepper

FOR THE CLAMS:

20g butter

2 tablespoons extra virgin olive oil

1 banana shallot

1 clove of garlic, crushed to a paste

250ml white wine

400g clams

200ml double cream

5g chopped fresh flat-leaf parsley

sea salt and freshly ground black pepper

200g samphire, to serve (asparagus would also work well)

Put the butter and oil for the cod into a frying pan and place over a medium heat. Once the butter stops foaming and starts to smell nutty, add the cod to the pan, skin side down. Baste the top of the fish with the butter and oil and cook for 5 minutes.

While the cod is cooking put the butter and oil for the clams into a saucepan, together with the shallot, place over a gentle heat and cook for 5 minutes to soften. Add the garlic and stir through for 90 seconds.

Flip the cod to cook the other side for 1 minute, then remove the fish and allow to rest.

Add the white wine to the pan and turn up the heat. As it boils, slide in the clams in one quick movement and put the lid on to capture the steam. Shake the pan to make sure the clams cook evenly. After 3 minutes, they should all be open, at which point add the double cream, parsley and some seasoning. If any clams remain closed after cooking, discard.

Lower the heat and continue to cook the clams for 3 minutes.

Meanwhile, bring a pan of salted water to the boil.

Plunge the samphire into the boiling water for 2 minutes, then drain. Divide between two plates, top with a cod fillet and pour the creamy clams on top.

Pan-fried Mackerel with Kimchi

SERVES 2

FOR THE MACKEREL:

2 tablespoons extra virgin olive oil

a knob of butter

2 mackerel, butterflied and skin scored

2 tablespoons Korean chilli flakes (gochugaru)

4 spring onions

1 teaspoon sesame seeds

1 lime, juice only

FOR THE SIDE SALAD:

100g mooli radish, cut into matchsticks

5 spring onions, shredded

1 cucumber, cut into matchsticks

a pinch of salt

½ teaspoon rice wine vinegar

½ teaspoon mirin

quick kimchi (see p.327), to serve

Put all the ingredients for the side salad into a small bowl. Mix well and leave to one side.

Put half the oil and the butter for the mackerel into a large frying pan and place on a medium heat. Add one mackerel, skin side down. (It may want to curl, so have a spatula handy to press down on it.) Cook for 3 minutes. Sprinkle half the chilli flakes over the flesh before flipping the fish and cooking for another minute.

Remove the fish from the heat and repeat with the other mackerel.

Serve, with the kimchi and side salad.

Monkfish Curry

SERVES 2

FOR THE CURRY BASE:

2 tablespoons extra virgin olive oil

1 onion, diced

3 cloves of garlic, roughly chopped

3cm piece of ginger, roughly chopped

2 red chillies, roughly chopped

20g roughly chopped fresh coriander

2 teaspoons turmeric

1 teaspoon yellow mustard seeds

1 teaspoon ground cumin

1 teaspoon ground coriander

½ teaspoon asafoetida

FOR THE CURRY:

2 tablespoons ghee

400ml coconut milk

300g monkfish fillet, cut into 2.5cm cubes (halibut or cod would also work well)

200g spinach

50g cherry tomatoes

sea salt and freshly ground black pepper

coconut flakes, toasted, and coriander leaves, to serve

This couldn't be quicker for a mid-week dinner. Put all the ingredients for the curry base into a mini-chopper or food processor and blitz to a rough paste.

Put the ghee for the curry into a large pan and, when hot, add the curry base and cook for 5 minutes over a gentle heat, stirring continuously to stop anything catching and burning.

Pour in the coconut milk and simmer for 10 minutes until the sauce has reduced and thickened. Add the monkfish, spinach and tomatoes and poach in the sauce for 5 to 7 minutes, until the monkfish is cooked.

To serve, season with salt and pepper, and garnish with the coconut flakes and coriander.

Delicious with a portion of nutty cauliflower rice (see p.330).

Pan-fried Scallops with Cauliflower Mash and Griddled Leeks

SERVES 2

FOR THE SCALLOPS:

10g butter

2 tablespoons extra virgin olive oil

6 rashers smoked bacon

10 scallops

1 lemon, juice only

sea salt and freshly ground black pepper

FOR THE MASH:

1 small cauliflower, broken into florets

50g butter

2 tablespoons extra virgin olive oil

sea salt and freshly ground black pepper

FOR THE GRIDDLED LEEKS:

20g butter

1 tablespoon extra virgin olive oil

12 baby leeks

¼ of a nutmeg, grated

First, make the mash. Bring a pan of water, with a steamer in it, up to the boil. Put in the cauliflower florets and steam for about 10 minutes, then tip into a colander to steam dry and leave to one side.

After 5 minutes, tip into a food processor and, with the motor running, add the butter, oil and some salt and pepper. Blitz until it is silky smooth, then transfer to a saucepan and put on a low heat to keep warm.

Heat a skillet over a medium heat and put the oil and butter for the leeks into it. Grate the nutmeg over the top and turn every now and again for 10 minutes, or until soft.

Put the butter and oil for the scallops into another frying pan, together with the bacon, and place over a high heat. Fry the bacon until crisp, then drain on a piece of kitchen paper. Add the scallops to the pan. Try not to move them or peep at them for 2 minutes (this will give them a beautiful caramelized crust), then flip to cook for another 2 minutes.

To serve, put a spoonful of the mash in the centre of a plate and top with the scallops and some butter from the pan. Put the leeks on the side and crumble the crispy bacon over them. Eat straight away.

Grandma's North Indian Chicken Curry

SERVES 2

4 tablespoons extra virgin olive oil

1 tablespoon ghee

1 large onion, finely chopped

4cm piece of ginger, finely chopped

3 cloves of garlic, finely chopped

1 tablespoon natural yogurt

400g chicken thighs, boned and chopped into chunks

2 teaspoons ground coriander

1 teaspoon garam masala

1 teaspoon freshly ground black pepper

1 teaspoon ground ginger

½ teaspoon turmeric powder

2 cloves

3 green chillies, finely chopped

5 large tomatoes, chopped

a pinch of salt

1 teaspoon balsamic vinegar

2 tablespoons chopped fresh coriander, a drizzle of extra virgin olive oil and 4 tablespoons natural yogurt, to serve

Put the oil and ghee into a large pan and place over a medium heat. Add the onion and ginger and cook for 8 to 10 minutes, until the onion starts to turn golden brown. Add the garlic and cook, while stirring, for another minute. Once the garlic has become aromatic, add the yogurt and stir to coat the onion mix before adding the chicken.

Add all the spices, mix well and cook for 2 minutes, then add the chillies and tomatoes.

Once the tomatoes have started to break down and are coating the chicken pieces, cover and simmer for 6 to 8 minutes. It should now look like a thickened sauce. Add the salt and the balsamic vinegar.

Cook for a further 6 to 8 minutes, or until the chicken is cooked, stirring continuously.

To serve, divide between two bowls and garnish with coriander and a drizzle of olive oil. Eat with cauliflower rice (see p.320) or mixed green vegetables (see p.325) and some natural yogurt.

Chicken Schnitzel with Sauerkraut

SERVES 2

FOR THE CHICKEN SCHNITZEL:

2 large chicken breasts, skin removed

1 large egg

100g ground almonds, sieved

50g Parmesan cheese, finely grated

2 teaspoons paprika

sea salt and freshly ground black pepper

40g butter

4 tablespoons extra virgin olive oil

FOR THE SAUERKRAUT:

500g white cabbage

2 tablespoons sea salt

If you fancy making your own sauerkraut, it is really easy – you just need to plan ahead. Using a mandolin or food processor, shred the cabbage as finely as you can and place in a large mixing bowl. Scatter with the salt, then massage together to start breaking it down. Do this for a minute or two, give your hands a rest, then do it for another minute or two. You should notice a growing pool of juice at the bottom of the bowl.

Take a 1-litre sterilized airtight jar or container and place some of the cabbage into the base. Using the end of a sterilized rolling pin, gently tamp it down, then add more cabbage and repeat. You want as little air as possible, to reduce the risk of any harmful bacteria developing. Pour in any leftover juices. Seal the jar and put it somewhere that isn't too cool and is out of direct sunlight.

Each day, release the gas that forms in the jar. If any foam appears on top of the juice, remove it. You could try the sauerkraut after a week but, as with all things fermented, it will be better the longer you leave it – or buy some fresh sauerkraut, if you can't wait!

To make the chicken schnitzel, lay a chicken breast just off centre on a large piece of baking paper. Fold the paper over and, with a rolling pin, bash the chicken breast until it is just under 1 centimetre thick. Repeat with the other breast.

Next, get two shallow bowls. Crack the egg into one and lightly beat. Mix the almonds, Parmesan, paprika and salt and pepper in another. Pat the chicken breasts dry with kitchen paper, then dip and turn them, one after the other, into the egg, then dip them into the almond mix. Make sure all the flesh is well covered.

Put the butter and oil into a large frying pan and place over a medium heat. Add the chicken and fry on each side for 4 to 5 minutes, or until the chicken is cooked through. You want the crumbs to go crisp and golden brown, but not to burn, while still cooking the chicken all the way through.

Serve each chicken breast with a pile of sauerkraut and some green vegetables.

Spatchcocked Chicken with Spiced Yogurt Marinade

SERVES 4 TO 6

1 chicken, approximately 1.8–2kg in weight, spatchcocked

FOR THE MARINADE:

250ml natural yogurt

2 tablespoons dried oregano

2 tablespoons paprika

1 tablespoon cayenne pepper

2 teaspoons chipotle chilli flakes (or regular chilli flakes)

1 teaspoon turmeric

1 lemon, juice only

sea salt and freshly ground black pepper

4 tablespoons extra virgin olive oil, to serve

To spatchcock the chicken, place it on a chopping board, breast side down. With a sharp pair of scissors, starting at the cavity and working towards the neck end, snip up each side of the chicken's backbone, then discard it.

Turn the chicken over and open it out, coaxing it, using a little pressure on the breastbone to make it lie flat.

Line a roasting tin with baking paper.

To make the marinade, put all the ingredients into a small bowl and mix until well combined.

Put the chicken into the baking tin, skin side up, and pour the marinade over it. With your hands, rub the marinade all over the chicken, on both sides. Cover the tin with cling film and refrigerate for 2 to 3 hours.

Heat the oven to 200°C/180°C fan. Put the chicken on the middle shelf for an hour, and turn halfway through.

Check the chicken is cooked before serving – all the flesh should be opaque, the juices should run clear when a knife is inserted into the thickest part of the leg and it should be hot through.

Serve with a salad, a cabbage slaw (see p.328), or broad beans with Parmesan (see p.326) – whatever takes your fancy.

Jerk Chicken Cauliflower Pizza

SERVES 2

FOR THE PIZZA BASE:

1 cauliflower, blitzed to cauliflower rice

2 tablespoons psyllium husk

1 tablespoon dried oregano

1 egg, lightly beaten

1 tablespoon extra virgin olive oil

FOR THE JERK CHICKEN:

2 chicken breasts

2 tablespoons jerk seasoning

1 tablespoon extra virgin olive oil

FOR THE TOPPING:

2 tablespoons tomato purée

2 ripe tomatoes, sliced

½ a red pepper, sliced

½ a yellow pepper, sliced

½ a green pepper, sliced

1 onion, sliced

fresh basil leaves

1 mozzarella cheese, torn into small chunks

2 tablespoons Parmesan cheese, grated

some rocket, and a drizzle of extra virgin olive oil, to serve

Preheat the oven to 200°C/180°C fan.

Heat a large frying pan over a medium heat and put the cauliflower into the dry pan. Keep stirring as it starts to cook. You don't want it to take on too much colour, but you need it to lose some of its moisture content so it makes a good base. This will take about 10 minutes. It should be around a quarter smaller in volume when it's ready.

Tip the cauliflower into a large mixing bowl while it's still steaming, and add the other ingredients for the pizza base. Mix well to distribute the egg.

Line two baking sheets with non-stick baking paper and brush with a little oil. Take half of the mix for the pizza base and drop it on to the tray, spreading it into a flat round – you don't want any holes or gaps. Repeat with the other baking sheet.

Place in the hot oven and cook for 20 to 25 minutes.

While the base is cooking, take the chicken breasts and rub them with the jerk seasoning and oil. Heat a griddle and cook each side for 6 to 7 minutes, or until cooked through. This will vary, depending on the shape and thickness of the meat. Set aside and slice when it has cooled a little.

Meanwhile, the edges of the pizza bases will be starting to brown and the bottom will be starting to dry out. After the first 20 minutes, remove the trays from the oven and carefully peel off the baking paper (minding your hands on the hot trays; a palette knife can be useful). Flip over to cook on the other side. Return to the oven and cook for a further 15 to 20 minutes, or until the middle is starting to colour and feels dry to the fingertips.

Take the bases out of the oven and increase the heat to 220°C/200°C fan. Spread half the tomato purée over each base, then layer with the rest of the toppings, finishing by dotting the cheese in and around to hold it all together.

Return the trays to the oven for 8 to 10 minutes. The peppers should just be starting to soften and the cheese to melt.

Serve with a big heap of rocket and a drizzle of oil.

Roast Aubergines with Feta, Herbs and Yogurt Dressing

SERVES 2

2 large aubergines, halved lengthways

3 tablespoons extra virgin olive oil, plus extra for drizzling

1 teaspoon pumpkin seeds

sea salt and freshly ground black pepper

FOR THE DRESSING:

100g natural yogurt

100g Greek yogurt

1 avocado, destoned and chopped

1 jalapeño pepper, deseeded and chopped

1 lemon, juice only

sea salt and freshly ground black pepper

120g feta cheese, crumbled, 60g walnuts, crumbled, 5g chopped fresh oregano leaves, 5g chopped fresh thyme leaves, and 1 teaspoon sesame seeds, to serve

Preheat the oven to 190°C/170°C fan. Line a medium-sized roasting tin with baking paper.

With a sharp knife, score the flesh of the aubergine to make a diamond pattern, being careful not to go through the skin. Brush the flesh with some of the oil, then drizzle with the rest. Scatter with the pumpkin seeds and season.

Cook in the oven for 20 minutes, then rotate the tray, adding a little more olive oil if the aubergines look as if they are drying out. Cook for another 20 minutes, or until the flesh is very soft all the way through.

While the aubergines are cooking, make the dressing by putting all the ingredients into a jug and whizzing together with a stick blender. If you want a looser dressing, add a tablespoon or two of water. Season and set to one side.

Divide the aubergines between two plates, add some dressing in blobs and scatter with the feta, walnuts, herbs and sesame seeds. Finish with a drizzle of oil.

Pumpkin, Mushroom and Sage Butter Courgetti

SERVES 2

FOR THE PUMPKIN:

½ a small pumpkin, peeled and cut into chunks

3 tablespoons extra virgin olive oil

sea salt and freshly ground black pepper

FOR THE MUSHROOMS:

50g butter

2 tablespoons extra virgin olive oil

200g chestnut mushrooms, thinly sliced

2 cloves of garlic, finely grated

5g chopped fresh sage

FOR THE COURGETTI:

1 tablespoon extra virgin olive oil

a knob of butter

2 large courgettes, spiralized

extra virgin olive oil, 20g Parmesan cheese shavings and a handful of pumpkin seeds, to serve

You will need: a spiralizer

Preheat the oven to 200°C/180°C fan.

Place the chunks of pumpkin on a lined baking sheet, drizzle with the extra virgin olive oil and season. Roast in the oven for 20 to 25 minutes until the pumpkin is soft all the way through. Take out of the oven and set to one side.

Place the butter and olive oil for the mushrooms in a wok over a medium high heat, until the butter has melted. Add the mushrooms and quickly flip to cover them in the butter and oil and get them cooking quickly. Cook for around 5 minutes, flipping every 30 seconds or so.

They should be taking on a lovely golden-brown colour. Add the garlic, sage and pumpkin and toss together. Tip into a large bowl and return the wok to the heat.

Put the oil and butter for the courgetti into the wok and add the spiralized courgettes. Toss them over a high heat for 2 to 3 minutes. You want them to be just starting to soften. Add the rest of the vegetables and toss together to combine.

To serve, divide between two bowls, drizzle with some oil and scatter with the Parmesan and pumpkin seeds.

Vegetable Curry

SERVES 2

1 medium sweet potato, washed, skin on

1 tablespoon ghee

4 tablespoons extra virgin olive oil

5 large tomatoes, chopped

4cm piece of ginger, finely chopped

2 green chillies, finely chopped

1 clove of garlic, finely chopped

200ml coconut milk

1 small aubergine, cut into 2cm pieces

½ a cauliflower, broken into bite-size pieces

1 tablespoon garam masala

½ a head of broccoli, broken into bite-size pieces

100g green beans, topped and tailed and cut into 2cm pieces

1 lemon, juice only

sea salt

4 tablespoons natural yogurt, to serve

Bring a pan of salted water up to the boil and carefully drop in the sweet potato. Boil for 15 to 20 minutes, or until you can insert a skewer easily. Once it is cooked, drain the hot water and mash, skin and all, and put to one side.

Put the ghee and extra virgin olive oil into a frying pan and place over a medium heat. Add the tomatoes, ginger and chillies and cook for 10 minutes, stirring every couple of minutes, until the tomatoes soften into a thick sauce.

Add the garlic and stir for 1 minute. Then add the mashed sweet potato and the coconut milk and stir to mix. Add the aubergine and simmer for 10 minutes, then add the cauliflower and garam masala. Turn the heat down low and cover the pan with a lid. Cook for 5 minutes before adding the broccoli and green beans.

Simmer for another 5 minutes until all the vegetables are al dente. Season with the lemon juice and a pinch of salt.

Serve with a spoonful of yogurt and a salad.

Low-carb Courgette Pizzas

SERVES 2

FOR THE BASE:

4 large courgettes, grated

½ teaspoon sea salt

1 egg, lightly beaten

50g ground almonds

50g Parmesan cheese

FOR THE TOMATO SAUCE:

2 tablespoons extra virgin olive oil

10g butter

1 small onion, finely chopped

1 teaspoon tomato purée

3 cloves of garlic, finely chopped

1 green chilli, finely chopped

½ teaspoon dried oregano

½ teaspoon dried basil

½ teaspoon dried thyme

1 x 400g tin of chopped tomatoes

1 teaspoon balsamic vinegar

FOR THE TOPPING:

basil leaves

1 mozzarella cheese

50g goat's cheese

4 chestnut mushrooms, sliced

1 red onion, thinly sliced

50g baby spinach, 50g rocket, 2 tablespoons extra virgin olive oil, and freshly ground black pepper, to serve

Preheat the oven to 190°C/170°C fan.

Place the grated courgettes in a large mixing bowl with the salt and massage together to start breaking them down. Leave for 5 minutes, then tip the courgettes into a clean towel and wring them out over the sink to get rid of any excess liquid. You don't want a wet pizza base, so this is very important.

Rinse and dry the bowl, return the courgettes to it, add the other ingredients for the base, and mix well. Line two baking sheets with non-stick baking paper and grease lightly with some extra virgin olive oil.

Tip out half of the mix on to each tray and shape into a round. Put the trays in the oven and cook for 20 to 25 minutes.

While the base is cooking, make the tomato sauce. Put the oil and butter into a medium-sized saucepan and place over a medium heat. When the butter has melted, tip in the onion and cook for 5 to 6 minutes, until it starts to soften. Add the tomato purée and cook for 2 minutes, until it becomes slightly darker in colour, then add the garlic, chilli and dried herbs. Stir for a minute, then pour in the tomatoes and the balsamic vinegar. Bring up to the boil, then simmer for 25 to 30 minutes.

Flip the courgette bases over after the first 20 to 25 minutes and return to the oven for 15 minutes. By then, the tomato sauce should be thick enough to spread over the base.

Top with the basil leaves, mozzarella and goat's cheese, mushrooms and red onion, and return to the oven for 10 minutes.

Serve with a handful of baby spinach and rocket leaves on top, a good glug of extra virgin olive oil and a twist of fresh pepper.

Sides

Green Salad

The best thing about a green salad is that it goes with everything. You want it to be crisp and crunchy to add texture to your meal.

SERVES 2

FOR THE SALAD, CHOOSE BETWEEN:

cos
romaine
frisée
iceberg
green and red chicory
radicchio
little gem
lollo rosso
oak leaf
red chard

spinach
rocket
watercress

FOR THE VINAIGRETTE:

4 tablespoons extra virgin olive oil
2 tablespoons apple cider vinegar
1 teaspoon Dijon mustard
½ a clove of garlic, crushed to a paste
sea salt and freshly ground black pepper

You can try substituting the apple cider vinegar for red or white wine vinegar; the Dijon for wholegrain or English mustard; the garlic for a spice like warm, earthy turmeric or chilli flakes. The variations are literally endless – so experiment.

Mixed Bean Salad

SERVES 2

PICK FROM A SELECTION OF
BEANS, TO INCLUDE AT LEAST 3
OF THE FOLLOWING:

60g runner beans

60g stringless helda beans

60g green beans, topped
and tailed

60g sugar snap peas

60g mangetouts

60g French beans

60g dwarf beans

4 tablespoons extra virgin
olive oil

sea salt and freshly ground
black pepper

OPTIONAL TOPPINGS:

30g toasted flaked almonds *or*

2 tablespoons poppy seeds *or*

½ a lemon, zest and juice *or*

30g pumpkin and sunflower
seeds *or*

½ teaspoon turmeric and ½
teaspoon cayenne pepper

Trim the beans, if needed. If the beans are quite large, you may wish to slice them into bite-size pieces.

Bring a saucepan of water to the boil, with a steamer basket on top. Place the beans in the steamer for 4 to 5 minutes, until al dente.

Drain and toss in a bowl with the olive oil, seasoning and your choice of topping.

Mixed Green Vegetables

SERVES 2

PICK FROM A SECTION OF
VEGETABLES TO INCLUDE AT
LEAST 3 OF THE FOLLOWING:

80g broccoli (tenderstem, purple
sprouting or regular)

80g spring greens

80g cabbage (sweetheart
or savoy)

60g kale

60g cavolo nero

60g green beans, topped
and tailed

60g runner beans

6 Romanesco cauliflower florets

2 tablespoons extra virgin
olive oil

10g butter

sea salt and freshly ground
black pepper

Steam the vegetables for 5 to 7 minutes. Drain into a colander.

Put the oil and butter into a large frying pan, place over a medium heat
and tip in the vegetables. Coat in the butter and season with salt and
pepper.

Try grating in a clove of garlic or adding a spoon of harissa, if you want
even more flavour.

Broad Beans and Parmesan

SERVES 2

200g baby broad beans

3 tablespoons extra virgin olive oil

½ a small clove of garlic, finely grated

20g Parmesan cheese, grated

5g chopped fresh mint leaves

½ a lemon, zest and juice

Bring a pan of salted water to the boil. Put in the baby broad beans and boil for 3 minutes.

Drain the beans and run under cold water for a minute or two to stop them cooking any further. Pop them into a mixing bowl. Add the oil, garlic, Parmesan, mint, lemon zest and a squeeze of lemon juice to taste.

Quick Kimchi

This will make more than you need for any single recipe, but it will keep fermenting and growing in flavour, so store and use as required.

1 Chinese cabbage, cut into 2cm slices

200g mooli radish, cut into matchsticks

1 bunch of spring onions, halved lengthways and shredded

2 tablespoons sea salt

3 tablespoons Korean chilli paste (gochujang)

3 tablespoons rice wine vinegar

2 tablespoons mirin

1 tablespoon fish sauce

4 cloves of garlic, finely grated

3cm piece of ginger, finely grated

Place the cabbage, mooli and spring onions in a mixing bowl and sprinkle with the salt. Use your hands to gently massage and squeeze the vegetables. Do this for 4 to 5 minutes, until they begin to soften and release some of their water.

Tip into a colander and rinse thoroughly to remove the salt. Pat dry in a clean tea towel and return to the mixing bowl.

Put the remaining ingredients into a separate bowl and mix together. Add to the cabbage, mooli and spring onions and mix together well, to coat everything with the spicy paste. Transfer the kimchi to a sterilized airtight container and pack down. Pop the lid on and leave, out of the fridge, to begin the fermentation overnight.

It will be ready to enjoy the next day, but it can be kept in the fridge for about a fortnight. The flavours will continue to develop and strengthen the longer it is left to ferment – experiment with how strong you like it for future batches.

Cabbage Slaw

SERVES 2

¼ of a red cabbage, very thinly sliced

¼ of a white cabbage, very thinly sliced

½ a red onion, very thinly sliced

5g roughly chopped fresh coriander leaves

2 tablespoons extra virgin olive oil mayonnaise

1 lime, juice only

sea salt and freshly ground black pepper

The easiest way to slice the vegetables is to use a mandolin; otherwise, slice the vegetables as thinly as you can with a very sharp knife.

Put all the ingredients into a large mixing bowl, mix well and set it to one side for 20 minutes to let the flavours mingle. If you like more of a kick, add a little more lime.

Quick Pickles

SERVES 2

½ a cucumber, cut into 3mm slices

1 onion, halved and cut into 3mm slices

¼ of a cauliflower, broken into small florets

50g sea salt

125ml apple cider vinegar

50ml water

1 teaspoon peppercorns

1 teaspoon coriander seeds

1 teaspoon mustard seeds

¼ teaspoon turmeric

Put the cucumber, onion and cauliflower into a mixing bowl and add the salt. Leave for half an hour, then massage gently for 1 minute before rinsing well under cold water to remove all the salt. You don't want to break the vegetables up – just coax some liquid loss. Put to one side.

Put all the remaining ingredients into a saucepan and bring to the boil. Add the rinsed cucumber, onion and cauliflower to the pan and cook for about 3 minutes. Transfer everything to an airtight container and leave to one side; an hour or two is perfect. These pickles will be crisp and crunchy and packed full of flavour.

Vegetable Rice

SERVES 2

½ a cauliflower, broken into florets, *or* ½ a head of broccoli, broken into florets, *or* 3 courgettes, cut into chunks

2 tablespoons extra virgin olive oil, plus a drizzle for cooking

a knob of butter

To make any of the vegetable rice options, the key thing is to preserve the texture of the vegetable and not let it go to mush.

Put the chosen vegetable into a food processor and quickly pulse on and off, on and off, until it is broken down into rough 'grains'. Be careful not to overdo it.

Put a small drizzle of oil into a large frying pan and spread around the base with a piece of kitchen paper, to prevent the vegetables from sticking. Turn the heat up high. Add the vegetable of choice and cook, stirring briskly, for 3 to 5 minutes. It will steam and reduce in size. Some water may release into the bottom of the pan, especially with the courgette, but just allow this to cook off.

The cauliflower will start to go a light golden brown – this will make it taste more nutty. Broccoli rice is softer in consistency, and the courgette a little smaller in grain and usually the softest of the three. All are delicious with any of the lunch and dinner recipes.

Serve immediately.

Pancetta Brussels Sprouts with Whole Almonds

SERVES 2

2 tablespoons extra virgin olive oil

40g pancetta

200g Brussels sprouts, halved

30g blanched almonds

1 clove of garlic, finely grated

2 tablespoons extra virgin olive oil and 1 tablespoon balsamic vinegar, to serve

Put the oil and pancetta into a wok and place over a medium heat. Once the fat from the pancetta has begun to melt, add the Brussels sprouts and almonds and toss together. Cook like this, shaking and tossing the ingredients in the wok, for 6 to 8 minutes. Add the garlic and toss for another minute.

To serve, tip into a serving dish and drizzle with the oil and vinegar.

Punjabi Salad

SERVES 2

1 large onion, diced
1 large tomato, diced
½ a cucumber, diced
1 tablespoon extra virgin olive oil

sea salt and freshly ground black pepper
1 lemon, juice only

Put the onion, tomato and cucumber into a mixing bowl. Drizzle with the oil and season to taste. Squeeze the lemon juice over everything, and mix well to bring it all together.

Indian-style Mixed Vegetables

SERVES 2

1 tablespoon ghee

1 head of broccoli or cauliflower, chopped

100g green beans, topped and tailed and chopped into small pieces

1 tablespoon garam masala

sea salt and freshly ground black pepper

2 tablespoons extra virgin olive oil, to serve

Put the ghee into a wok and place over a high heat. Add all the vegetables and cook for 5 minutes, shaking and tossing the pan to keep them moving and cooking evenly.

Lower the heat and stir in the garam masala and some salt and pepper.

Cover with a lid and continue cooking for 10 minutes, shaking the wok occasionally.

To serve, drizzle with extra virgin olive oil.

Tray-baked Roast Vegetables

PICK FROM A SELECTION OF
VEGETABLES, TO INCLUDE AT
LEAST 4 OF THE FOLLOWING:

6 cauliflower florets

6 broccoli florets

80g Brussels sprouts

60g shallots

1 red onion, cut into 6 wedges

8 asparagus spears

1 head of fennel, sliced

1 large courgette, cut into chunks

1 pepper, sliced (red, orange, yellow or green)

1 aubergine, sliced into rounds

1 head of garlic, broken into cloves

4 tablespoons extra virgin olive oil

sea salt and freshly ground black pepper

Preheat the oven to 200°C/180°C fan.

Line a large roasting tray with baking paper.

Put the vegetables of your choice into the tray and cover with the oil and some salt and pepper. Put the tray into the hot oven for 15 minutes, then stir, turning them over, to make sure they roast evenly.

Return the tray to the oven for another 15 minutes, then serve.

Leek and Courgette Gratin

SERVES 2

2 tablespoons extra virgin olive oil

40g butter

3 leeks, ends trimmed and outer layer discarded, sliced lengthways and into 4mm-thick slices

2 large courgettes, topped and tailed, sliced lengthways and into 4mm-thick slices

3 cloves of garlic, finely grated

1 tablespoon English mustard

250ml double cream

1 teaspoon paprika

10g roughly chopped fresh thyme leaves

50g Parmesan cheese, grated

50g ground almonds

sea salt and freshly ground black pepper

Preheat the oven to 200°C/180°C fan.

Put the oil and butter into a large-based sauté pan over a medium heat. Add the leek and cook for 3 minutes. Next, add the courgettes, and cook for 2 minutes. Add the garlic, and cook for 1 minute, stirring continuously to prevent it burning.

Stir through the mustard and double cream and bring to a simmer.

Add the paprika and thyme leaves and mix well. Leave to cool gently while you grease a 1.5-litre, deep ovenproof dish with a little butter. Once ready, pour the leeks and courgettes into the dish.

Put the Parmesan, ground almonds and some salt and pepper into a small bowl and sprinkle it over the leek and courgette mix. Place the tray into the hot oven and cook for 20 to 25 minutes, until golden brown and bubbling nicely.

Cabbage Thoran

SERVES 2

2 tablespoons coconut oil

1 banana shallot, finely chopped

1 green chilli, finely chopped

½ teaspoon turmeric

1 teaspoon cumin seeds, toasted

1 teaspoon mustard seeds

1 small sweetheart cabbage, shredded

100g desiccated coconut, toasted

chilli flakes, to serve

Put the oil into a wok and place over a high heat. Once hot, add the shallot and chilli and cook for 2 minutes, stirring frequently. Add the spices and cook for another minute.

Once everything is really aromatic, add the cabbage and toss with the spices until well coated. As the cabbage is so finely cut, this won't take long to cook. Keep it moving in the pan for 2 minutes before adding the coconut and tossing through.

Serve immediately.

Notes

2. The Pioppi Diet: A Healthcare Manifesto

1. Lustig, R. H., 'Processed Food – An Experiment That Failed', *JAMA Pediatrics* (2017), 171(3): 212–14; doi:10.1001/jamapediatrics.2016.4136.

2. Brownell, K. D., 'Thinking Forward: The Quicksand of Appeasing the Food Industry', *PLoS Medicine* (2012), 9(7): e1001254; doi:10.1371/journal.pmed.1001254.

3. Malhotra, Aseem, 'It's Time to Ban Junk Food on Hospital Premises', *British Medical Journal* (2013), 346: f3932.

4. Rechel, Bernd et al., 'Ageing in the European Union', *Lancet*, vol. 381, issue 9874, 1312–22.

5. Hex, N., et al., 'Estimating the Current and Future Costs of Type-1 and Type-2 Diabetes in the United Kingdom, including Direct Health Costs and Indirect Societal and Productivity Costs', *Diabetes Medicine* (July 2012), 29 (7): 855–62; doi: 10.1111/j.1464-5491.2012.03698.x.

6. http://static.latribune.fr/463077/etude-morgan-stanley-impact-diabete-sur-l-economie-mondiale.pdf.

7. Briggs, A. D. M., et al., 'Overall and Income-specific Effect on Prevalence of Overweight and Obesity of 20% Sugar-sweetened-drink Tax in UK: Econometric and Comparative Risk Assessment Modelling Study', *British Medical Journal* (2013), 347: f6189.

8. Frieden, T. R., 'A Framework for Public Health Action: The Health Impact Pyramid', *American Journal of Public Health* (2010), 100: 590–95.

9. Credit Suisse Research Institute, 'Fat: The New Health Paradigm' (2015), 76.

10. Scott, H., et al., 'Infographic: Tomorrow's Doctors Want to Learn More about Physical Activity for Health', *British Journal of Sports Medicine* (2017), 51: 624–5.

11. NYU Langone Survey presentation to American College of Cardiology's 64th Annual Scientific Session, March 2015.

4. Why Pick On Sugar?

1. https://www.ucl.ac.uk/news/news-articles/0914/160914-Experts-call-for-radical-rethink-on-free-sugars-intake.

2. Lustig, Robert H., 'Sickeningly Sweet: Does Sugar Cause Type-2 Diabetes? Yes', *Canadian Journal of Diabetes* (2016), vol. 40, issue 4, 28–6.

3. Lustig, R. H., Schmidt, L. A. & Brindis, C. D., 'The Toxic Truth about Sugar', *Nature* (2012), 487: 27–9.

4. Basu, S. et al., 'The Relationship of Sugar to Population-level Diabetes Prevalence: An Econometric Analysis of Repeated Cross-sectional Data', *PLoS ONE* (2013), 8: e57873.

5. Yang, Q., et al., 'Added Sugar Intake and Cardiovascular Diseases Mortality among US Adults', *JAMA Internal Medicine* (2014), 174(4): 516–24; doi:10.1001/jamainternmed.2013.13563.

6. Lustig, R. H., et al., 'Isocaloric Fructose Restriction and Metabolic Improvement in Children with Obesity and Metabolic Syndrome', *Obesity* (Silver Spring) (2016), 24(2): 453–60; Epub, 26 October 2015.

5. Saturated Fat Does Not Clog the Arteries

1. Credit Suisse Research Institute, 'Fat: The New Health Paradigm' (2015), 76.

2. Harcombe, Z., Baker, J. S. & Bruce, B., 'Food for Thought: Have We been Giving the Wrong Dietary Advice?', *Food and Nutrition Sciences* (2013), vol. 4, no. 3: 240–244.

3. de Souza, R. J., et al., 'Intake of Saturated and Trans Unsaturated Fatty Acids and Risk of All-cause Mortality, Cardiovascular Disease, and Type-2 Diabetes: Systematic Review and Meta-analysis of Observational Studies', *British Medical Journal* (2015), 351: h3978.

4. Chowdhury, R., et al., 'Association of Dietary, Circulating, and Supplement Fatty Acids with Coronary Risk: A Systematic Review and Meta-analysis', *Annals of Internal Medicine* (2014), 160(6): 398–406; doi: 10.7326/M13-1788.

5. Schwingshackl, L. & Hoffmann, G., 'Dietary Fatty Acids in the Secondary Prevention of Coronary Heart Disease: A Systematic Review, Meta-analysis and Metaregression', *British Medical Journal Open* (2014), 4: e004487.

6. Harcombe, Z., et al., 'Evidence from Randomised Controlled Trials Did Not Support the Introduction of Dietary Fat Guidelines in 1977 and 1983: A Systematic Review and Meta-analysis', *Open Heart* (2015), 2(1); doi: 10.1136/openhrt-2014-000196.

7. Malhotra, A., 'Saturated Fat is Not the Major Issue', *British Medical Journal* (2013), 347; doi:10.1136/bmj.f6340.

8. Mozaffarian, D., Rimm, E. B. & Herrington, D. M., 'Dietary Fats, Carbohydrate, and Progression of Coronary Atherosclerosis in Postmenopausal Women', *American Journal of Clinical Nutrition* (2004), 80: 1175–84.

6. Cholesterol: Friend or Foe?

1. Anderson, K. M., Castelli, W. P. & Levy, D., 'Cholesterol and Mortality: 30 Years of Follow-up from the Framingham Study', *JAMA* (1987), 257(16): 2176–80; doi:10.1001/jama.1987.03390160062027.

2. Schatz, Irwin J., et al., 'Cholesterol and All-cause Mortality in Elderly People from the Honolulu Heart Program: A Cohort Study', *Lancet* (2001), vol. 358, issue 9279, 351–5.

3. Ravnskov, U., et al., 'Lack of an Association or an Inverse Association between Low-density-lipoprotein Cholesterol and Mortality in the Elderly: A Systematic Review', *British Medical Journal Open* (2016), 6: e010401.

4. DuBroff, Robert, 'Cholesterol Paradox: A Correlate Does Not a Surrogate Make', *Evidence-based Medicine* (March 2017), 22(1): 15–19; doi:10.1136/ebmed-2016-110602.

5. Champeau, R., 'Most Heart Attack Patients' Cholesterol Levels Did Not Indicate Cardiac Risk', UCLA Newsroom, 2009, http://newsroom.ucla.edu/portal/ucla/majority-of-hospitalizedheart-75668.aspx.

6. Da Luz, P. L., et al., 'High Ratio of Triglycerides to HDL-Cholesterol Predicts Extensive Coronary Disease', *Clinics* (Sao Paulo, Brazil) (2008), 63(4): 427–432; doi:10.1590/S1807-59322008000400003.

7. Ramsden, C. E., et al., 'Re-evaluation of the Traditional Diet–Heart Hypothesis: Analysis of Recovered Data from Minnesota Coronary Experiment (1968–73)', *British Medical Journal* (2016), 353: i1246.

8. http://www.thennt.com/nnt/statins-for-heart-disease-prevention-with-known-heart-disease/.

9. http://www.thennt.com/nnt/statins-for-heart-disease-prevention-without-prior-heart-disease/.

10. http://www.prescriber.co.uk/news/clarity-needed-true-benefits-risks-statins/.

11. http://www.nytimes.com/1987/07/14/science/cholesterol-debate-flares-over-wisdom-in-widespread-reductions.html?pagewanted=all.

7. The Root Cause of Heart Disease:
Insulin Resistance and Inflammation

1. Facchini, F. S., et al., 'Insulin Resistance as a Predictor of Age-related Diseases', *Journal of Clinical Endocrinology and Metabolism* (August 2001), 86(8): 3574–8.

2. Eddy, D., et al., 'Relationship of Insulin Resistance and Related Metabolic Variables to Coronary Artery Disease: A Mathematical Analysis', *Diabetes Care* (2009), 32(2): 361–6; doi: 10.2337/dc08-0854.

3. https://www.escardio.org/Journals/E-Journal-of-Cardiology-Practice/Volume-8/TG-HDL-ratio-as-surrogate-marker-for-insulin-resistance.

4. Rothberg, M. B., 'Coronary Artery Disease as Clogged Pipes: A Misconceptual Model', *Circulation: Cardiovascular Quality and Outcomes* (2013), 6: 129–32.

5. Malhotra, Aseem, 'The Whole Truth about Coronary Stents: The Elephant in the Room', *JAMA Internal Medicine* (2014), 174: 1367–8.

6. Sargent, R. P., Shepard, R. M. & Glantz, S. A., 'Reduced Incidence of Admissions for Myocardial Infarction Associated with Public Smoking Ban: Before and After Study'

[with commentary by T. Pechacek and S. Babb], *British Medical Journal* (2004), 328: 980–83 (24 April).

7. Barnoya, B. & Stanton, A., 'Cardiovascular Effects of Second-hand Smoke', *Circulation* (2005), 111: 2684–98, doi:10.1161/CIRCULATIONAHA.104.492215.

8. Estruch, R., et al., 'PREDIMED Study Investigators. Primary Prevention of Cardiovascular Disease with a Mediterranean Diet', *New England Journal of Medicine* (2013), 368: 1279–90.

9. Restrepo, Brandon J., et al., 'Denmark's Policy on Artificial Trans Fat and Cardiovascular Disease', *American Journal of Preventive Medicine* (2016), vol. 50, issue 1, 69–76.

10. https://bmcmedicine.biomedcentral.com/articles/10.1186/s12916-017-0791-y.

11. http://casagutier.com/wp-content/uploads/2016/04/Simopoulos-omega3-review-2004.

12. Simopoulos, A. P. & Di Nicolantonio, J. J., 'The Importance of a Balanced ω-6 to ω-3 Ratio in the Prevention and Management of Obesity', *Open Heart* (2016), 3: e000385; doi: 10.1136/openhrt-2015-000385.

13. http://www.telegraph.co.uk/news/health/news/11981884/Cooking-with-vegetable-oils-releases-toxic-cancer-causing-chemicals-say-experts.html.

14. http://www.cochrane.org/CD006742/HTN_benefits-of-antihypertensive-drugs-for-mild-hypertension-are-unclear.

15. Blackburn, E. H. & Epel, E. S., 'Too Toxic to Ignore', *Nature* (2012), 490: 169–71.

16. Manchanda, S. C., et al., 'Yoga Reduces Blood Pressure in Patients with Prehypertension', Association of Physicians of India (July 2000), 48(7): 687–94.

8. Type-2 Diabetes is Carbohydrate-intolerance Disease

1. https://www.ucsf.edu/news/2012/08/12501/almost-half-type-2-diabetes-patients-report-acute-and-chronic-pain.
2. http://archive.jsonline.com/watchdog/watchdogreports/effects-of-diabetes-drugs-dubious-b99398554z1-286482971.html.
3. Spence, Des, 'Bad Medicine: The Way We Manage Diabetes', *British Medical Journal* (2013), 346: f2695.
4. Malhotra, A., Maruthappu, M. & Stephenson, T., 'Healthy Eating: An NHS Priority. 'A Sure Way to Improve Health Outcomes for NHS Staff and the Public', *Postgraduate Medical Journal*, published online first: 16 November 2014, doi:10.1136/postgradmedj-2014-133103.
5. Feinman, R. D., et al., 'Dietary Carbohydrate Restriction as the First Approach in Diabetes Management: Critical Review and Evidence Base', *Nutrition* (2015), 31: 1–13.

9. Stop Counting Calories and Stop Snacking

1. Kekwick, A. & Pawan, G. L., 'Calorie Intake in Relation to Body-weight Changes in the Obese', *Lancet* (1956), 271: 155–61.
2. Strohacker, K. & McFarlin, B., 'Influence of Obesity, Physical Inactivity, and Weight Cycling on Chronic Inflammation', *Frontiers in Bioscience* (2010), E2: 98–104; doi:10.2741/e70.
3. Fildes, A., et al., 'Probability of an Obese Person Attaining Normal Body Weight: Cohort Study Using Electronic Health Records', *American Journal of Public Health* (2015), 105: e54–e59.
4. Wing, R. R., et al., Look AHEAD Research Group, 'Cardiovascular Effects of Intensive Lifestyle Intervention in

Type-2 Diabetes', *New England Journal of Medicine* (2013), 369: 145–54; doi:10.1056/NEJMoa1212914.

10. The Physical Activity Obesity Myth: You Can't Outrun a Bad Diet

1. Luke, A. & Cooper, R. S., 'Physical Activity Does Not Influence Obesity Risk: Time to Clarify the Public Health Message', *International Journal of Epidemiology* (2013), 42: 1831–6; doi:10.1093/ije/dyt159.
2. https://www.ncbi.nlm.nih.gov/pubmed/21449785.
3. 'Exercise – The Miracle Cure. Report from the Academy of Medical Royal Colleges' (February 2015), http://www.aomrc.org.uk/.
4. Moore, S. C., et al., 'Leisure-time Physical Activity of Moderate to Vigorous Intensity and Mortality: A Large Pooled Cohort Analysis', *PLoS Medicine* (2012), 9: e1001335.
5. Hall, S. A., et al., 'Sexual Activity, Erectile Dysfunction, and Incident Cardiovascular Events', *American Journal of Cardiology* (2010), 105(2): 192–7; doi:10.1016/j.amjcard.2009.08.671.

11. Movement is Medicine

1. https://www.ncbi.nlm.nih.gov/pubmed/21618162.
2. https://www.ncbi.nlm.nih.gov/pubmed/21450618.
3. http://www.cell.com/cell-metabolism/fulltext/S1550-4131(17)30099-2.
4. http://bjsm.bmj.com/content/early/2014/07/30/bjsports-2013-093342.short?g=w_bjsm_ahead_tab.
5. de Brito, L.B.B., et al., 'Ability to sit and rise from the floor as a predictor of all-cause mortality', European Journal of Preventive Cardiology, vol.21,7:pp.892-898.

12. Stress
(Further References)

https://www.ncbi.nlm.nih.gov/pubmed/28058238.

Sahin, E. and DePinho, R. A., 'Linking Functional Decline of Telomeres, Mitochondria and Stem Cells during Ageing', *Nature*, 2010, 464:520–28.

https://www.ncbi.nlm.nih.gov/pmc/articles/PMC5209646/.

'Sedentary Behavior, Physical Activity and Cardiorespiratory Fitness on Leukocyte Telomere Length'.

Conclusion: individuals who are physically active, engage in less sedentary behaviour and have higher levels of cardiorespiratory fitness have the longest leukocyte telomere length (LTL).

https://www.ncbi.nlm.nih.gov/pubmed/25944259.

'Leisure-time, Screen-based Sedentary Behavior and Leukocyte Telomere Length: Implications for a New Leisure-time, Screen-based Sedentary Behavior Mechanism'.

The results of this study revealed that greater leisure-time, screen-based sedentary behaviour is associated with shorter LTL.

https://www.ncbi.nlm.nih.gov/pubmed/25970659.

'Movement-based Behaviors and Leukocyte Telomere Length among US Adults'.

Greater engagement in movement-based behaviours is associated with reduced odds of being in the lowest LTL tertile.

14. Intermittent Fasting

1. Moror, T., et al., 'Effects of Eight Weeks of Time-restricted Feeding (16/8) on Basal Metabolism, Maximal Strength, Body Composition, Inflammation, and Cardiovascular Risk Factors in Resistance-trained Males', *Journal of Translational Medicine* (2016), 14: 290; https://translational-medicine. biomedcentral.com/articles/10.1186/s12967-016-1044-0, doi:10.1186/s12967-016-1044-0.

18. Aseem and Donal's Top-Ten Foods

1. http://www.ncbi.nlm.nih.gov/pubmed/17513403.

Acknowledgements

This book is a tribute to all those doctors, scientists, health activists, journalists and friends whose tireless work, help and support has help make this book come to fruition for the sole purpose of helping millions improve their health for the better:

Professor Robert Lustig, Professor Simon Capewell, Dr Richard Feinman, Professor Grant Schofield, Dr Caryn Zinn, Dr Trudi Deakin, Gary Taubes, Nina Teicholz, Dr Zoe Harcombe, Sam Feltham, Professor Zbys Fedorowicz, Dr Deborah Cohen, Professor Rita Redberg, Dr Pascal Meier, Dr Stephen Phinney, Professor Timothy Noakes, Karen Thomson, Sir Richard Thompson, Professor David Haslam, Dr Shamil Chandaria, Sami Inkinen, Dr Sarah Hallberg, Dr Andreas Eenfeldt, Dr Rangan Chatterjee, Dr Jason Fung, Lord Ian Mccoll, Andy Burnham, Luciana Berger, Denis Campbell, Edward Malnick, Jonathan Ungoed-Thomas, Warwick Harrington, Ben Spencer, Andrew Greggory, Katie Gibbons, Ivor Cummins, Dr Ted Naiman, Dr Maryanne Demasi, Dr Ross Walker, Luciana Berger, Baroness Shami Chakrabarti, Amanda Platell, Jeremy Vine, Professor Chris Ham, Dr Chaand Nagpaul, Dr Fiona Godlee, Dr David Unwin, Dr James Di-Nicolantonio, Dr Frank Lipman, Dr Mark Hymann, Dr Clare Gerada, Emma Sinclair, Dale Pinnock, Giles Sheldrick, Cristina Earle, Dr Victor Montori, Dr Partha

ACKNOWLEDGEMENTS

Kar, Dr Esther Van Zuuren, Professor Hanno Pijl, Carole
Stone, Richard Lindley, Rob Yates, Anushka Asthana, Dr
Zafar Iqbal, Karim Khan, Professor Peter Brukner,
Damon Gameau, Louise Knoop O'Neill, Professor James
McCormack, Dr JS Bamrah, Professor Terence Stephenson,
Professor Mike Rayner, Dr Ben Maruthappu, Anahad O'
Connor, Katia Michael, Jamie Oliver, Gurinder Chadha,
Dorrit Mousaieff, Christine Cronau, Dr Rod Tayler, Lisa
Kelly, Adam Brimelow, Adam Bullimore, Kay Burley,
Eamonn Holmes, Stephen Dixon, Professor Dame Sue
Bailey, Professor Sir Muir Gray, Alexandra Phillips, Dr
Cristina Romete, Keith Vaz, Namita Panjabi, Katie Silver,
Shaminder Nahal, Artemis Simopoulos, Sarah Knapton,
Emma Alberici, Rory Robertson, Sarah Wilson, Professor
Nita Farouhi, Thea Jourdan, Rosamund Urwin, Susanna
Reid, Karen Aston, Simon Stevens, Alastair Henderson,
Professor David Newman, Pete Evans, Zena Tuitt, Wayne
Richmond, Ivor Cummins, Dr Jeffrey Gerber, Max
Lugavere, Dr Laurie Rauch, Andre Oelofse, Tiny
Laubscher, Yolanda Barker, Marek Polaszewski, Antonio
Morinelli, Angelo Morinelli, Gerry Chile, Stefano Pisani,
Sami Inkinen, Lucy Johnston, Paul Gallagher, Esther
Rantzen, Laura Donnelly, Jules Stenson, Ed Vanstone,
Ted Lane, Dr John Abramson, Dr Uffe Ravnskov, Dr
Michel De-Lorgeril, Professor Sherif Sultan, Dr David
Ludwig, Anahad O'Connor, Dr Neville Wellington, Dr
Philip Mills.

A special thanks to Dale Pinnock, Dr Trudi Deakin
and Dr Caryn Zinn for their input and helpful comments
for the Top-Ten Foods chapter.

Index

Recipe Index